Professional Development and Management for Therapists

An Introduction

Professional Development and Management for Therapists

An Introduction

Editors:

Elizabeth Murray MBA, BA, MCSP

and

Jill Simpson MSc, MCSP

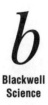

**Blackwell
Science**

© 2000 by
Blackwell Science Ltd
Editorial Offices:
Osney Mead, Oxford OX2 0EL
25 John Street, London WC1N 2BL
23 Ainslie Place, Edinburgh EH3 6AJ
350 Main Street, Malden
  MA 02148 5018, USA
54 University Street, Carlton
  Victoria 3053, Australia
10, rue Casimir Delavigne
  75006 Paris, France

Other Editorial Offices:

Blackwell Wissenschafts-Verlag GmbH
Kurfürstendamm 57
10707 Berlin, Germany

Blackwell Science KK
MG Kodenmacho Building
7-10 Kodenmacho Nihombashi
Chuo-ku, Tokyo 104, Japan

The right of the Author to be identified as
the Author of this Work has been asserted
in accordance with the Copyright, Designs
and Patents Act 1988.

First published 2000

Set in ITC Century and produced by Gray
Publishing, Tunbridge Wells, Kent
Printed and bound in Great Britain by
Biddles Ltd,
Guildford and King's Lynn

The Blackwell Science logo is a
trade mark of Blackwell Science Ltd,
registered at the United Kingdom
Trade Marks Registry

DISTRIBUTORS

  Marston Book Services Ltd
  PO Box 269
  Abingdon
  Oxon OX14 4YN
  (*Orders*: Tel: 01235 465500
         Fax: 01235 465555)

USA
  Blackwell Science, Inc.
  Commerce Place
  350 Main Street
  Malden, MA 02148-5018
  (*Orders*: Tel: 800 759 6102
         781 388 8250
       Fax: 781 388 8255)

Canada
  Login Brothers Book Company
  324 Saulteaux Crescent
  Winnipeg, Manitoba R3J 3T2
  (*Orders*: Tel: 204 837-2987
       Fax: 204 837-3116)

Australia
  Blackwell Science Pty Ltd
  54 University Street
  Carlton, Victoria 3053
  (*Orders*: Tel: 03 9347 0300
       Fax: 03 9347 5001)

A catalogue record for this title is
available from the British Library

ISBN 0-632-05107-8

Library of Congress
Cataloging-in-Publication Data is available

For further information on
Blackwell Science, visit our website:
www.blackwell-science.com

Contents

Contributors

Sarah Burnard
Director, Practices Made Perfect, Brighton

Val Glenny
Team and Organisational Development Consultant

Pat Oakley
Senior Consultant and Director, Practices Made Perfect, Brighton

Penelope Robinson
Director, Professional Affairs Department, Chartered Society of
Physiotherapy, London

Jeanette Standring
Senior Lecturer, School of Physiotherapy, Manchester Royal
Infirmary

Hélène Wilkinson
Senior Specialist, Practices Made Perfect, Brighton

Preface

The National Health Service (NHS) has undergone rapid and extensive change since the early 1990s and this is set to continue well into the twenty-first century. It remains the major employer of the whole range of Professions Allied to Medicine (PAMs). However, no longer do therapy students enter a workplace where one employer is very similar to another, where the terms and conditions of their employment are similar across the country, where their career pathway is clearly mapped out or where they are guaranteed a job for life. Never before has the work of therapists been so demanding mentally and physically, or so much expected of individuals in so many ways. This is equally true for PAMs who have worked in their fields for some time. This book aims to identify and clarify management and career issues which impact on the working lives of therapy and PAMs staff. It is particularly targeted at students close to graduating, newly qualified or training-grade PAMs.

Although the book aims to consider issues which will impact on therapists whatever their working environment, it focuses largely on the NHS both as the major provider of health care in the UK and as the biggest employer of PAMs. The topics covered by the book were determined via some focus-group work carried out by the editors with their own junior staff. In such a rapidly changing environment as exists in today's NHS, it is not atypical to have current trends or 'flavours of the month'. The text strives to achieve a balance between covering the key issues which may underpin these whilst providing information which is up to date at the time of writing.

The book's contents will be of equal relevance to students graduating into many PAMs, including newly qualified physiotherapists, occupational therapists, speech and language therapists, orthoptists, dieticians and radiographers. However, its main focus is on the first three of these, i.e. the therapy professions. Some of its contents will also be of value to other students or new graduates in wider health professional groups such as pharmacy, clinical psychology, nursing and medicine. In many of the contexts described, the terms PAM and therapist are used interchangeably.

Chapter 1 aims to provide an overview of the young therapist or PAM working in today's health-care environment. It introduces many of the issues to be explored further in the other chapters. In particular, it highlights the issues likely to face new therapists when making the transition to working life, some important considerations for therapists in managing themselves and their career, and some background on key, relevant management theory, considered to be of value to PAMs.

Chapter 2 outlines the organisation of the NHS and the effect of recent and ongoing changes. How these will shape the different organisations within the NHS in the future and the expectations that may be placed on therapists are surmised. Being aware of the development of PAMs is important in understanding how services and professions have reached the stage they are at today; it also gives some pointers on how things may look in the future. This is developed throughout Chapter 3, including an overview of the implications for individual career development.

Within any relationship between employees and employer there will be expectation on both sides. Chapter 4, 'Getting Started in a Job', provides information on the recruitment process, what to look out for when considering where to work and the assistance that should be given to new recruits by an organisation. This knowledge should aid therapists in deciding on the appropriate organisation to match their expectations.

All organisations rely on good teamwork to work effectively. Therapists have always naturally worked with others to provide holistic care to patients. Chapter 5, 'Working with People', investigates how teams are formed, the roles and responsibilities taken by people within them and what is required for a team to be successful. These factors are crucial for effective interdisciplinary working both now and in the future.

Chapter 6 outlines the main legislation which governs or guides therapists' practice, especially in the NHS. This is considered to be important information which may not be fully covered in undergraduate training. Chapter 7 also covers issues which are crucial to working life but are not normally addressed within training courses. The principles of personnel policies and procedures should be understood and may be particularly important to those changing jobs between different organisations.

Managing one's own career pathway will be an important aspect of working life. Chapter 8, 'Career and Personal Development', gives an overview of the issues involved in doing this in today's health-care world. It also outlines how tools such as appraisal, mentorship and reflective practice can enhance a career and ensure continued professional development.

All therapists are encouraged to hold membership of their professional bodies, which may have a number of roles; in some cases this is mandatory. Newly qualifying therapists should understand the roles of these bodies and how they can help and support them. Chapter 9, 'Professional Organisations', aims to help the reader to appreciate the roles and uses of a range of professional bodies.

Although many therapists choose to start their career and continue to work within the public-sector organisations within the UK, recently more are deciding to work with different employers. The final chapter of this book aims to highlight the key issues for those considering employment outside the NHS, largely within the private or voluntary sector.

At the time of writing, no text addresses the above issues and it is hoped that the book is a worthwhile addition to the libraries of PAMs' training schools and service departments, as well as of value to aspiring, individual clinicians.

Acknowledgements

The publisher wishes to thank the following for their permission to reproduce copyright material in Chapter 5: page 61: M. Belbin, *Team Roles at Work*, p. 23, Butterworth Heinemann, Oxford. Page 62: précis of 'Informational influence and normative influence' (pp. 205–207) by Colin Fraser from *Introducing Social Psychology* edited by Henri Tajfel and Colin Fraser (Penguin Books, 1990) copyright © Henri Tajfel and Colin Fraser; reproduced by permission of Penguin Books Ltd. Page 64: Jon R. Katzenbach and Douglas K. Smith, *The Wisdom of Teams: Creating the High-Performance Organization*, Boston: Harvard Business School Press, 1993, pp. 20–23. Page 66: G. Morgan, *Images of Organization* (p. 149), copyright © G. Morgan, reprinted by permission of Sage Publications. Page 67: K. Back and K. Back, *Assertiveness at Work*, second edition, pp. 89 and 95, Ken & Kate Back Ltd. Page 70: N. Hayes, *Successful Team Management* (pp. 194–195), International Thomson Publishing, 1977.

The editors wish to acknowledge the contributions made by the following people to Chapter 10: Mrs S Nesbitt, Physiotherapy Manager, The Alexandra Hospital, Cheadle, Manchester; Miss E Carrington, Foreign Affairs Officer, Chartered Society of Physiotherapy; Mr K Harvey, Physio First, Towchester.

Chapter 1
An Introduction: Working Life, Today's Health Service and Management

Introduction

Entering the field of work for the first time or moving to a new organisation can be a daunting undertaking for any member of the Professions Allied to Medicine (PAMs). The majority of newly qualifying PAMs still look towards the National Health Service (NHS) as their first employer, although this is declining. In 1994 as many as 27.6% of newly qualified PAMs chose not to work in the NHS (NHSE North West, 1994). As a result of the reorganisations within the NHS over the past 20 years, gone are the days when PAMs, especially therapists, could be familiar with the structure and organisation of the service they joined within the NHS. In the 1970s and early 1980s there was a similar pattern to each therapy service, including how it was organised and managed. Following the NHS reforms at the beginning of the 1990s, many different management arrangements for PAMs services have emerged. There has also been a drive to improve the efficiency and effectiveness of services provided. Different management structures and organisational arrangements have different influences on the way in which PAMs work. For today's clinicians, it is important that the various factors that create these influences are considered before therapists either embark on or, through a promotion, develop their career in any organisation.

The topic of management may seem irrelevant to therapists at the beginning of their career or when newly promoted to a senior level. This book aims to provide such PAMs with basic information about management and how it relates to them. The book will also introduce therapists to issues and concepts which may be relevant to them as individuals, to the management of their career and to working in an ever-changing environment. It also addresses some of the issues associated with how therapists relate to colleagues and the overall management process.

This chapter provides an introduction to some of the issues and concepts covered in this book. The chapter begins by describing some of the factors to be considered when choosing where to work and getting a job. This is followed by an outline of some of the major differences between student and working life, and an overview of changing and developing careers. The second half of the chapter addresses relevant management theory: its definition, what managers do, management styles, motivation and an overview of how individuals fit within the business of organisations.

Choosing where to work

Most therapists, certainly for the first year or two after qualifying, will choose to work in a large organisation, probably a hospital and probably within the NHS. The following paragraphs summarise a few key issues which may be of particular consideration to the new or young PAM beginning their working life in such an environment.

Working within a large campus, such as a major teaching hospital, may be attractive to those who have gained experience of this at university and who enjoy busy surroundings. However, if this is not an individual's preferred atmosphere, it may be better to seek employment in a smaller organisation such as a District General Hospital or Community Trust. Whilst larger organisations may appear threatening and impersonal this is not necessarily the case, and they often provide a very stimulating working environment. Smaller organisations are often perceived to be friendly, welcoming and warm, but this may be counterbalanced by more rigid approaches which do not encourage innovation. These are general statements about perceptions and should be taken as such. The only way that therapists can really understand their preferred working environment is to visit organisations and talk to the staff who already work there. Only from information gathered in this way can a real picture be painted of what a particular organisation is like.

In many NHS Trusts PAMs professional groups are beginning to be managed as a single unit or directorate. It is important that staff within individual professions are aware of the influence that different management arrangements may have on their career development. PAMs working and being managed together in an organisation, rather than a disparate groupings, often makes improvements for the whole.

Ultimately, therapists must decide which type of organisation fits with their expectations and consider the factors that the organisation will require in its employees. At this point, some graduates may prefer more autonomy, in which case private practice may be more appropriate. More details of this and other types of work are given in Chapter 10.

Getting a job

Therapists are extremely fortunate. At present, within the UK, there are generally more vacancies than there are qualified people to fill them. This is not the same for all health professional groups.

Over their first 2–3 working years, most managers expect a frequent turnover of junior staff and this is not deemed to be negative. It allows individuals to develop laterally through experiences of different organisations, which can have a positive effect on their overall development. However, very frequent changes in job can have a negative effect, especially during the first few years of work. Such action can indicate lack of consistency, direction or satisfaction with a therapist's career. It is generally recognised that it takes approximately 18 months following qualification for therapists to consolidate their learning and achieve a sense of achievement and direction from their work. It is also recognised that in the early years of their career, therapists have greater mobility and are willing to move around for the right job. Later, when they adopt family or other responsibilities, their ability to move is restricted; this limits their choices of places to work and possibly also the field or area available for them to work in.

Taking responsibility for work

Making the transition from student life to beginning a working career can be quite a striking change. As a student, most therapists take responsibility only for themselves, concerned mainly with completing assignments or study plans. On clinical placements there is close supervision and support from qualified clinicians.

Upon qualifying and commencing work as a therapist, staff are accountable for their own actions as well as being responsible for the guidance of others. Therapists' actions are now likely to impact on many other people, not least patients. PAMs may be required to supervise assistants and possibly students, and work in a variety of teams such as with PAMs in other local therapy departments (possibly through rotational schemes), with nurses and doctors on wards or within the community.

Of particular importance to clinicians is their prime responsibility to patients: therapists are accountable for what they do with patients. This transition may not be easy. Personal learning takes on new and different dimensions, where learning from training is applied and developed. Rather than seeing them as negative, colleagues appreciate new staff recognising their limitations and asking for assistance when required. Senior staff are well aware that undergraduate education provides a sound basic knowledge but further training is needed to become a

competent practitioner. In addition, professional codes of conduct emphasise that clinicians should not practise in areas in which they are not
competent without adequate supervision.

Real learning begins when therapists start work and are able to apply
the theories and techniques learned as a student. Through experience
gained from practice, clinicians learn the theories and methods to use in
particular circumstances. Some of this learning will be acquired through
direct clinical practice, some will be learning from others, particularly
senior staff, and some from mistakes. Whilst the latter must be avoided,
it is almost inherent that some will be made along the way. They should
not be a source of great worry and it is helpful for a colleague to act as
a mentor in learning from the situation.

Another marked difference from student activity that newly qualified
staff will encounter is the pace and volume of work expected in today's
workplace. Over the past few years the health service has strived to
increase efficiency, demanding more work in less time. It can be argued
that time for learning and development has suffered as a consequence
of this. However, the introduction of clinical governance (see Chapter 2)
means that organisations must also ensure that staff are up to date with
the latest knowledge and implement evidence-based practice.

Career pathways

Changes in career patterns

A career may span as many as 40 years and, just as in life, a career will
move ever onwards with choices and milestones along the way. Traditionally, career progression has always been viewed vertically; that is,
progress meant movement upwards in hierarchical steps. The number of
opportunities for advancement in an upward direction varies amongst
occupations and organisations. In the past, PAMs could follow a fairly definite career pathway through the NHS, via the grading structures set out
in the Whitely Council agreements (see Chapter 7). With the flattening of
organisational structures over recent years, there are now fewer hierarchical steps; some perceive that their career has come to an end when
they reach a particular level and there are no specific opportunities for
advancement. Whilst some may continue to advance upwards, even outside their own occupation, others reach and remain at a certain level for
prolonged periods. Today, senior clinical therapists often perceive that
opportunities for vertical advancement have become restricted.

However, today's career must be seen as the ability to continue to grow
personally and not be solely viewed as progressively moving upwards
(Mayo, 1991). This philosophy is being expounded by all professional bodies in their statements on continuous professional development.

A career can be viewed in many different ways. Schein (1971) describes a career cycle, having external movement and reference points for how the internal career is experienced. A career can also have a functional dimension, which describes a special area of expertise. Schein (1971) indicates that this may mean very little vertical movement for those in a particular occupational group. Within the PAMs, it is possible to work across various clinical specialities through rotational schemes. These allow the development of different specialist skills and knowledge. It is also possible for an individual, having specialised in a particular area, to change or extend their field of expertise to something new. Whilst this would not necessarily mean vertical progression, it would be indicative of horizontal or lateral growth on a personal and professional level.

A career can also develop towards the core of a profession or organisation. This usually happens when an individual increases their knowledge base and receives recognition for this. They become a trusted staff or team member and acquire responsibility. This may be typical of some highly specialist senior clinicians; however, this is not always the case. Some clinicians remain on the periphery even though they grow vertically. Inner movement can be very meaningful, leading to special involvement and rewards such as access to exclusive information, and this type of growth should not be regarded as being 'stuck' in relation to career progression.

For therapists or PAMs, these dimensions of career progression can be depicted as an organisational cone (Fig. 1.1). The criteria for movement along each axis can be defined as:

- promotion for the vertical direction
- rotation for the horizontal direction
- acceptance as movement towards the centre (also horizontal in direction).

As a result of the increased importance of its employees to its success, an organisation may now have a strategy to help in managing the careers of its employees. Mayo (1991) defines such a strategy as 'the design and implementation of organisational processes which enable careers of individuals to be planned and acceptance managed in a way that optimises both the needs of the organisation and preferences and capabilities of individuals'.

Starting a career

As this book is aimed at newly qualified therapists or those aspiring to their first senior position, only the early stages of a career pathway (i.e. over the first few years) will be outlined. During this period, the career of therapists tends to follow a typical pathway; after this time, the career pathway is less predictable and can extend in many directions.

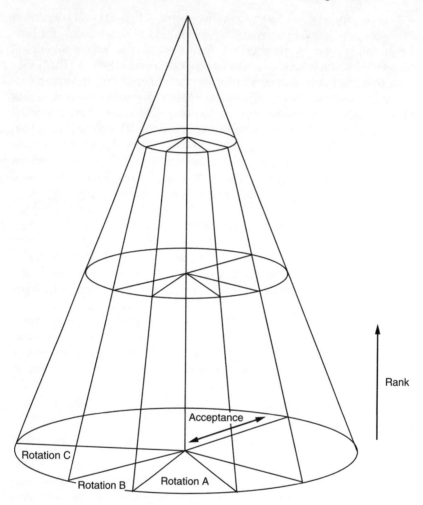

Fig. 1.1   Dimensions of career progression.

It is natural to have aspirations and ambitions for advancement. In the early years of working life, therapists will be greatly influenced by the qualities and experiences of senior colleagues with whom they have regular contact.

The first 10 years of a career are considered to be a period of learning, when knowledge is gained and skills are developed; theory is put into practice and experience gained. It may be felt that having chosen a particular profession a career pathway has been defined, and some may find it difficult to move outside the traditional routes for health-care professionals. However, the need for greater flexibility and blurring of professional roles in the new NHS will facilitate therapists' learning roles traditionally undertaken by others and allow a greater range of opportunities for career development in the future.

Employers are now attempting to attract staff by offering packages which include flexible hours and child care, which may allow individuals greater freedom to apply for posts in different areas. The current Government is shortly to launch a strategy on child care, and employers may offer other assistance with child-care costs through a voucher scheme, on-site crèche or information on the availability of local, high-quality child-care facilities.

The previous pages have described some aspects of the current environment in which therapists may find themselves working. The next few pages consider some of the more theoretical considerations associated with management and working in organisations.

What is management?

Understanding management will help to explain the integral link between therapists and the management process in any organisation. This will ensure that they work together to best effect. However, making sense of management is not easy.

Management can be viewed as an art, science, politics or magic (Watson, 1986). Managers have been referred to as 'those that get work done through others' or 'those who motivate people to achieve optimum performance'. Whichever view is taken, the most appropriate may vary depending on the individual manager and the type or level of role in which he or she operates. There are many definitions of management, including:

> ... to manage is to forecast and to plan, to organise, to command, to co-ordinate and to control (Fayol, 1949)

> ... running things properly (Mant, 1979)

> ... the co-ordination of human & material resources toward objective accomplishment (Kast & Rosenzweig, 1970)

> ... pulling things together and along in a general direction to bring about long-term organisational survival (Watson, 1986).

Staff may have their own ideas about what they perceive as management, which may or may not be based on previous experience. Despite much study, there does not appear to be much resemblance between what managerial work appears to be in practice and some of its traditional definitions.

Management was initially evaluated in the early twentieth century by F.W. Taylor, who tried to apply a 'scientific approach', particularly to ways of improving efficiency. He was responsible for the development of what are now known as 'time and motion studies'.

In the 1940s, a 'human relations' approach was developed with the work of Rensis Leikert and Douglas McGregor, who made the association between group behaviour in the work place and management styles to which they were subjected. This work demonstrated that people work best when their managers have genuine concern for their well-being.

One of the most influential attempts to illuminate managerial work is that of Mintzberg (1973). He identified 10 roles which he believed encompassed managerial work:

- interpersonal roles
  - (1) figurehead
  - (2) leader
  - (3) liaisor
- informational roles
  - (4) monitor
  - (5) disseminator
  - (6) spokesman
- decisional roles
  - (7) entrepreneur
  - (8) disturbance handler
  - (9) resource allocator
  - (10) negotiator.

Whilst these are the components of managerial work, there remains considerable variety in the extent to which they are present in different management jobs and the way in which they are dealt with by managers.

What do managers do?

Managers of PAM services will undoubtedly undertake the roles described by Mintzberg. However, with the present variation in structural arrangements within and between organisations, there are no specific rules regarding who or what level of individual will undertake certain roles. Some of the roles described above may be carried out by senior clinical staff in addition to or instead of managers. Regardless of who undertakes a role or how, in practice, it is carried out, every PAM service will have someone who fulfils the duties described by Mintzberg.

A manager of any of these services will act as a figurehead for the service or profession to higher levels of management within their own organisation as well as to other managers or agencies outside the organisation. Such a role will also involve the manager leading the PAM service and suggesting how the service should progress or change. Original management theories suggested that leaders were 'born not made', but a comparison of 100 studies looking at leadership traits showed only 5% of personal characteristics that are common throughout (IHSM/

Open University, 1991). It is not always the most charismatic people who are the most effective leaders. Peters & Waterman (1982) define leadership as 'being visible when things go awry, and invisible when they are working well. It is building a loyal team that speaks more or less with one voice'.

A PAMs manager will often act as a spokesperson, offering professional advice and liaising with other managerial colleagues. Well-developed communication and interpersonal skills are essential for this; managers of PAMs are often recognised for such abilities and are frequently used by their organisation to make links with other agencies, e.g. social services and voluntary agencies.

Managers play a significant role in dealing with information, monitoring the use of resources such as staff, equipment and budgets as well as monitoring service clinical activity, either in terms of numbers (e.g. outputs or contacts) or, more importantly, in terms of effectiveness. This aims to ensure good use of human resources. Managers have a key role in both developing their staff and monitoring the ways in which they work. This may necessitate corrective action, or changes in staff roles or tasks in order to meet service requirements (see Chapter 4, Clarifying the job).

Managers also play a role in disseminating information to their staff from higher levels of management and communicating with other managers within the organisation, in health authorities or other agencies.

Staff may also look to their manager for ideas or solutions to difficulties or problems or rely on them to suggest new ways of doing things; managers should make it easy for staff to approach them about such issues. A common method today is the 'open-door' policy, where staff can access a manager directly without appointment or having to go through others to obtain their permission. Managers can also facilitate staff access by their interpersonal skills and demonstrating understanding of the issues with which they are presented. Explanation of access arrangements to managers should be included within the induction process (see Chapter 4).

Finally, managers can be called upon to address situations of difficulty or dispute amongst staff or between staff and management. Although uncommon, this may result in the enactment of organisational grievance or disciplinary procedures, further details of which are given in Chapter 7.

The extent to which managers may undertake all of the roles outlined above will vary within organisations and the scope of the manager's responsibility. For example, the manager of a large therapy service with 100 staff is likely to have a greater sphere of control and influence than one who manages a small team of 10 staff.

Management styles

The manner in which a manager carries out the above roles may be important in staff's ability to work and function well. There are many styles of
implementing management roles. For example, a manager may have a
democratic approach, where he or she seeks views on issues from staff
and works with staff to determine solutions or answers. More *autocrat-
ic* managers may feel that through their experience and their role, they
are more able to make decisions or find solutions. In today's world, and
in general, the former approach is considered to be the more successful
method. Active staff participation in raising issues and problems and finding solutions usually leads to the most practical and acceptable end result.
However, as many managers will know, on occasions this approach is not
appropriate and they need to adopt a different style of management.
Managers are held accountable for the decisions that they make.

Throughout this book, some of the ways in which PAMs may relate to
their managers are explored in detail. The book also highlights some managerial areas where therapists should take personal responsibility for
either taking action or acquiring knowledge.

Motivation at work

As a career is likely to cover a long period, maintaining motivation and
interest in work is crucial to ensure job satisfaction. Some background
on motivation may help to enlighten therapists on how it can be attained
and retained throughout their career.

Every individual has needs. These range from the basic ability to exist
and survive, through feeling that they 'belong', to having a sense of growth.
The relative importance of these needs to individuals changes over time.
The needs can only be satisfied by attaining goals which arise from them
(e.g. food and shelter for continued existence, acceptance by colleagues
or family to belong, and status or recognition for growth). Behaviour is
aimed at attaining these goals; that is, goals motivate individual behaviour. Whether or not motivation is sustained depends on whether or not
we perceive the outcomes of our behaviour to be rewarded.

Much has been written about motivation. However, a theory commonly
considered is that of Herzberg. Herzberg identified two sets of factors
affecting motivation, described as 'satisfiers' and 'hygiene factors' (or 'dis-
satisfiers'). Satisfiers included sense of achievement, levels of responsibility, the content of the work and advancement. Responsibility was
deemed to be particularly important. Hygiene factors included workplace
conditions, salary levels and organisational policies. Herzberg postulat-
ed that *both* sets of factors were important, but it was the satisfiers that
actually motivated people.

It may be beneficial for therapists to reflect on these issues from time to time throughout their career. Factors that motivate will enhance performance in the workplace. It may be good for clinicians to seek or experience these factors, and managers should facilitate this. An example of this may be encouraging staff participation in managing change and decision making. Where staff have been able to influence decisions associated with changes, they have greater 'ownership' for the new circumstances and are more motivated to see them succeed.

Working in organisations

All organisations or businesses, from single-handed private practice to large organisations, should have clear objectives. This will include organisations considering future as well as current demands. In service industries, such as therapy services, the largest resource needed to meet these demands is skilled people. The aim of most employers in achieving their objectives is to ensure they have the right people with the right skills at the right time. Therefore, the appropriate recruitment, training and development of people are crucial for health organisations (and, within these, therapy services) to meet their objectives. However, how an organisation requires its staff to develop may not always match up with individuals' interests and aspirations. Subsequently, there may be a tension between staff and organisational development needs.

The development of people and organisations is extremely complex but it is important to understand that there is an interaction between the individual and their place of work over time (Schein, 1978). Both exist within a society and culture, each having its own set of beliefs, values and criteria for measuring success. As individuals, therapists enter their chosen profession based on their self-assessment, i.e. personal interests, key abilities and where they perceive opportunities for development. Other important factors, such as family and home life, will also influence this decision. Through the business and strategic planning process, organisations also undertake an assessment which contributes to a determination of objectives and, subsequently, what is required to achieve these. As highlighted previously, in service industries, this is largely people. However, in recruiting and developing people, organisations must take account of the wider needs and issues of employees. Traditionally, there was a view that employees should 'leave their personal lives at home'; now, however, most organisations and managers realise that only by understanding the need for and relationship between the various elements of employees' lives, can they optimise the potential of individuals. Thus, a careful balance has to be struck between providing individual employees with opportunities for rewarding work and career development, and the organisation obtaining effectiveness and efficiency in providing its services.

Summary

This book aims to expand on many of the issues raised above. This chapter has highlighted some of the issues likely to face new therapists when making the transition to working life. It should also give the reader, the new or young PAM, some sense of the inter-relationship between them and any organisation in which they work or plan to work. It has also raised some important considerations for therapists in managing themselves and their career, which should be carefully thought about from an early stage. Some background on key, relevant management theory, considered to be of value to PAMs, has also been described.

This first chapter has set the scene for the remaining chapters, which will consider many of the above issues in further detail.

References

Fayol, H. (1949) *General and Industrial Management.* Pitman, London.

IHSM/Open University. *Managing Health Services* (1991) Open University Press, Milton Keynes.

Kast, F.E. & Rosenzweig, J.E. (1970) *Organization and Management: A Systems Approach.* McGraw-Hill, New York.

Mant, A. (1979) *The Rise and Fall of the British Manager.* Macmillan, London

Mayo, A. (1991) *Managing Careers – Strategies for Organisations.* Institute of Personnel Management, London.

Mintzberg, H. (1973) *The Nature of Managerial Work.* Harper & Row, New York.

NHSE North West (1994) *Manpower Returns for the Professions Allied to Medicine.* NHSE North West.

Peters, T.S. & Waterman, R.H. (1982) *In Search of Excellence.* Harper & Row, New York.

Schein, E.H. (1971) The individual, the organisation and the career: a conceptual scheme. *Journal of Applied Behavioural Science* **7**, 401–26.

Schein, E.H. (1978) *Career Dynamics: Matching Individual and Organisational Needs.* Addison-Wesley, Wokingham.

Watson, T.J. (1986) *Management Organisation and Employment Strategy.* Routledge Kegan Paul, London.

Further reading

Crabtree, S. (1991) *Moving Up: A Practical Guide to Career Advancement for Managers, Consultants and Professionals.* Kogan Page, London.

Chapter 2
The Health-Care Business: An Overview

Introduction

Since its introduction in 1948, the National Health Service (NHS) has attempted to fulfil its broad objectives of providing comprehensive services to all, which are free at the point of delivery, and which are delivered at the time they are needed.

In organisational terms, the NHS is a bureaucracy, that is, an organisation characterised by rigid rules, with an organisational hierarchy and centralised decision making. Whilst having many advantages, some of the drawbacks of a bureaucracy include a certain amount of rigidity and difficulty in innovating and implementing organisational change quickly. In order to overcome some of these difficulties, there has been a number of key organisational reforms during the history of the service, as the NHS continued to refine its organisation and policy to meet the health needs of the population within its budgetary constraints.

This chapter describes the current structure of the NHS, resulting from the two most recent broad sets of reforms (in the late 1980s and in the 1990s, including the most recent changes introduced from 1997), its funding flows and government changes. It examines the implications for the services arising from the reforms and indicates the role of the various organisations within the structure. It also describes NHS corporate and business planning, and 'contracting' complexities. Finally, it highlights some of the key features of NHS therapy services and other organisations with which therapy services may interact.

The structure of the NHS: to 1997

The Department of Health

The arrangements described below relate to England; in Wales, health matters are dealt with by the Welsh Office Health Department; in Northern Ireland by the Department of Health and Social Services; and in Scotland by the Scottish Office.

In England, the Secretary of State for Health is a member of the cabinet of the government of the day and, as such, is an elected Member of Parliament. The Secretary of State for health is accountable to Parliament for every aspect of the service, and is responsible for the service as a whole; the Secretary of State's role involves setting the strategic direction for the service supported by the Department of Health.

The NHS Executive and the eight Regional Offices (ROs) in England form part of the Department of Health. The Executive is responsible for implementing NHS policy, managing the operation of the service and managing the funding.

Regional offices

The ROs are responsible for co-ordinating services at their individual local level. The eight regional offices in England are:

- Northern and Yorkshire
- Trent
- Anglia and Oxford
- North Thames
- South Thames
- South and West
- West Midlands
- North West.

The eight ROs co-ordinate the work of the integrated Health Authorities covered by each geographic region.

Health authorities

Each Health Authority is accountable to its host RO and is led by a Chairperson, appointed by the Secretary of State for Health. Until 1996, there were two types of HA, the Family Health Services Authority (FHSA) and the District Health Authority (DHA). The former was responsible for primary care and the latter for secondary care, mental health services and community care. In April 1996, FHSAs and DHAs merged into Health Authorities (HAs); on average, each HA is currently responsible for the care of approximately half a million people.

NHS Trusts

Hospitals and community services within the NHS are run as self-governing Trusts, each organisation being led by a Chairperson and a Board of Directors. Boards comprise both Directors of the Trust and non-executive members. The latter may be drawn from organisations within the local community, and may bring with them experience and knowledge from industries outside the NHS.

Trusts are accountable to the Secretary of State for Health and their host RO monitors their performance.

The 1989 reforms

The NHS reforms of 1989 introduced the concept of the 'internal market' to the NHS. In this model a notional health 'marketplace' was created, and some organisations being responsible for purchasing health care, with other parts of the service designated providers of care. Health Authorities and general practitioner (GP) fundholders were the main purchasers, whilst the providers were NHS Trusts and organisations outside the NHS arena, e.g. the voluntary and private sectors. Funds were designated to follow patients through their episodes of care; the concept of competition was introduced to encourage improvements in efficiency and effectiveness and increase responsiveness to patients' needs and demands.

GP fundholders were responsible for assessing the health needs of their local population and for purchasing the best possible care for them. The providers of care were given the freedom to manage their own budgets to provide services in the most effective way.

In this model both purchasers, and vicariously patients, had freedom to select the care they needed. Currently, the idea of competition has been reduced in favour of collaboration whilst, in essence, the marketplace remains unchanged (i.e. nominal purchasers and providers still exist).

NHS funding in the recent past

In order to appreciate the context in which the NHS operates it is important to understand how money flows into the service and how these funds are dispersed and translated into money to fund direct patient care.

Figure 2.1 indicates the passage of funds through the service up until 1997 and early 1998. Most of the funds used by the NHS are raised through the system of general taxation. The remainder is raised through other extraneous charges, such as prescriptions.

Whilst the Secretary of State is responsible for ensuring that the NHS operates within its financial limits, he or she is also responsible for trying to obtain the best deal possible from the service in securing funds from the Chancellor of the Exchequer. All government departments negotiate with the Chancellor for funds for their own particular departments.

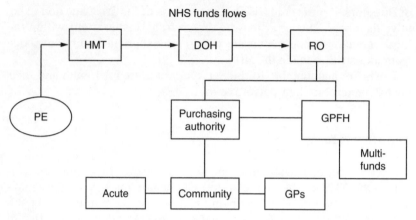

Fig. 2.1   Passage of funds through the NHS. GPFH, GP fundholders; DOH, Department of Health; RO, Regional Offices; HMT, Her Majesty's Treasury; PE, public expenditure pay round.

The Secretary of State for Health in this sense is in competition with his or her cabinet colleagues for what he or she considers to be a fair share of the funds that are available for the Chancellor to disperse to the possible sectors every year. The annual round of negotiation is known as the public expenditure pay round, and is part of the government's annual budget-setting cycle.

Once the Secretary of State for Health has secured finances for the coming year, these are then dispersed throughout the service, through the Department of Health and the NHS Executive, to ROs, Health Authorities and other purchasers. Up to this point funds have not reached the level where they may be dispersed to pay for direct patient care and, as such, this allocation may be seen as an overhead to the NHS. This is an important point because it will help to explain some of the rationale behind recent reforms that have attempted to reduce the cost of this overhead. For example, the reforms of the late 1980s and then of the 1990s resulted in a reduction in the number of Regions from 16 to eight and a reduction in the number of Health Authorities (from the merger of DHAs and FHSAs).

NHS Trusts, the provider organisations, have the freedom to decide the mix of staff that they wish to employ and the ways in which they wish to reward staff. The majority of Trust budgets is spent on staff salaries, approximately 80%, and the remainder may be classed as overheads, expenditure on non-clinical staff, heating, light, buildings, etc.

The latest reforms

The New NHS: Modern–Dependable (White Paper)

Some key themes recur throughout this White Paper, which was published in December 1997. They are as follows.

(i) First and foremost, the *abolition of the internal market*: the White Paper opposed the concept of the internal market, and promoted the concept of integrated care; the latter model will drive the NHS in the future. For example, NHS bodies are to have a new statutory duty of partnership placed on them, to ensure that different agencies work together for the 'common good'. In this context, the concept of 'competition' is replaced by one of 'collaboration'. Local Authorities, which provide Social Services, such as home helps, social work and occupational therapy, are also to be included in this initiative. [Social Services Departments (SSDs) of English Health Authorities are overseen by the Department of Social Services, whereas NHS bodies such as hospital Trusts and Health Authorities are overseen by the Department of Health.]

(ii) The introduction of *clinical governance*: the development of local and national quality standards, the setting up of new national bodies, such as the National Institute for Clinical Excellence (NICE) and the Commission for Health Improvement (CHI), and the bringing together of such important issues as risk management and continuing professional development, are all elements of the government's intention to make sure that clinical governance is a key priority for all care provider organisations.

These initiatives and developments are likely to be underpinned by emerging new legislation (the Civil Rights Bill) to ensure that a series of scandals involving substandard performance of clinicians resulting in patients' injuries and deaths (which were made public in 1997 and 1998) does not recur.

Other important themes include:

- the increased involvement of doctors, nurses and other clinicians in care planning and commissioning
- information technology supporting actual care delivery rather than being used only in administrative functions
- performance measurement of Trusts to be broader based than previously and to include assessment of health improvement, fair access to services, efficient and effective delivery of care, the patient/carer experience and the health outcomes of NHS care.

Some key implications of the White Paper

The new arrangements will mean changes in the role of existing agencies and the emergence of a new type of organisation: Primary Care Groups (PCGs). In the paragraphs below, these changes are examined and the new financial and accountability arrangements described in brief.

England

Health Authorities

The number of Health Authorities in England is set to decrease, and mergers between existing Health Authorities can therefore be expected. Their key role will be to develop a 3-year Health Improvement Programme in consultation with care providers, including with Local Authorities. They will also be responsible for monitoring its implementation.

The Health Improvement Programmes will represent the local strategy to deliver national targets. They will cover the health needs and the health-care requirements of the local population, encompassing both the public health efforts required by the various care partners (and not just the NHS bodies) and the way in which local services should be developed to meet them. They will also describe the range, location and investment required in local health services to meet the health needs of the local population.

Over time, it is envisaged that Health Authorities will relinquish their commissioning activities as PCGs increasingly take over this responsibility.

Health Authorities will also have a role in co-ordinating local workforce plans, and in co-ordinating information and information technology plans in their area.

NHS Trusts

NHS Trusts are to participate in the development of Health Improvement Programmes, which will set the framework for local service agreements with Health Authorities and the new PCGs. In particular, these service agreements will include quality measures. They will last for longer periods than the current annual contracts.

Legislation is to be drawn up to give Trusts a new duty for the quality of care. (The current principal statutory duties are financial.) Clinical governance, based on processes of quality improvements, the development of evidence-based practice and the monitoring of clinical performance, is to be introduced in all Trusts and overseen by a senior clinician.

Primary Care Groups

These will be groups of GPs (who will remain independent contractors), community nurses and other community staff. They will evolve from current schemes such as GP fundholding, total purchasing projects and locality commissioning GPs, and from Community NHS Trusts. They cover a population of around 100,000 patients.

PCGs will, in the first instance, be expected to contribute to the development of Health Improvement Programmes. They will then take devolved responsibility for managing the budget for health care in their locality as part of the Health Authority. As they mature, they will become freestanding bodies accountable to the Health Authority for commissioning care; finally, they will also be responsible for providing community health services in their area. Freestanding PCGs will become Primary Care Trusts (PCTs) and new legislation will provide for the establishment of this new status. PCTs may merge with all or part of existing Community NHS Trusts.

All PCGs will be expected to take on their full responsibility over time, but the rate of progress towards this target will depend on the pre-existing stage of development of GP commissioning in different areas. PCGs were established from April 1999.

PCGs and Trusts will be accountable to Health Authorities, including financially. They will have the freedom to deploy their resources within the framework of the Health Improvement Programme. They will have a single unified primary care budget, covering hospital and community health services and prescribing. These unified budgets were introduced from April 1999. There will also be a combined PCG and Health Authority management budget for each Health Authority area.

Health Authorities themselves will retain their statutory accountability to the NHS Executive, as will NHS Trusts. NHS Trusts will agree long-term service agreements with PCGs, around specific care areas.

Wales

The NHS Directorate for Wales represents the NHS Executive and, as such, fulfils some of the functions of ROs in England. Wales currently has five Health Authorities, which have similar commissioning and strategic responsibilities to their English counterparts. NHS Trusts have completed the process of being reconfigured, and Local Health Groups were introduced in Wales in April 1998.

Scotland

The Scottish office represents the NHS Executive. Fifteen Health Boards (12 mainland and three island boards) are directly accountable to the Scottish office. The Health Boards have a strategic, health-improvement, public-health and performance-management role.

The Boards are each served by NHS Trusts and proposals exist to decrease the number of Trusts in Scotland. The remaining Trusts will fall into two categories: Acute Hospital Trusts and PCTs.

There is also an intention to develop Local Health Care Co-operatives. These will be units within PCTs, responsible for populations of natural communities (25,000–150,000 people). They will be responsible for delivering and managing services for their local area. This structure will permit GPs to extend further their current primary care teams, thus providing a greater range of services directly to their patient population.

Northern Ireland

Currently, the Department of Health and Social Services and the Health and Social Services Executive are responsible for legislation, policy and strategy in relation to Health and Personal Social Services (HPSS) at regional level.

There are two chief groups within HPSS: commissioners and providers of services. The commissioners include four health and social service Boards and 171 GPFH units. The providers include 19 Health and Social Service Trusts, five Health and Social Service Agencies, and all the independent family health service clinicians.

In future, it is proposed that there will be one regional organisation responsible for management of HPSS and for strategy, policy and legislation: the new Department of Health, Social Services and Public Safety. It is also proposed that new Health and Care partnerships are developed, to assess health and social care needs and fulfil a commissioning and public health role; the partnerships will comprise several Primary Care Co-operatives at a local level.

Services will be provided by a mixture of integrated Health and Social Service Trusts, and by Health and Social Service Agencies. The latter currently provide diverse services, whilst the former provide integrated health and social care.

Other developments

Around the same time as the White Paper was published, two Green Papers (or consultation documents) were published: one (*Our Healthier Nation*) represents the first step towards a national health promotion strategy, and the other (*A National Framework for Assessing Performance*) proposes a framework against which NHS services are to be assessed in the future.

In *Our Healthier Nation*, national targets are set and proposal set out for consultation on how these might be achieved across the country and how success could be monitored. In *A National Framework for Assessing Performance*, emphasis is placed on Trusts' accountability to Health Authorities for their clinical performance, as well as their financial performance. Trusts and PCGs/PCTs will have to have mechanisms in place to ensure that they carry out their duties in relation to clinical governance.

Health Action Zones (HAZs) are recent initiatives (1997) resulting from funds released by the government. They promote the concept of effective multiagency working by tackling inequalities through promoting 'seamless service provision' for both health and other care agencies (e.g. Social Services, the voluntary sector). They aim to achieve benefits in areas of deprivation through innovative working. Examples include:

- collaboration between a Health Authority, NHS Trusts, voluntary organisations, the Local Authority and a Community Health Council in an area of economic deprivation and high mortality due to cancer and to coronary heart disease
- a project between different agencies to target unemployment in young males from ethnic minority groups, decreasing the death rate from strokes and heart disease, and improving mental health in the under-30s.

Corporate and business planning

The corporate and business planning process in the NHS is driven by the strategy for the service set by the Secretary of State for Health. Once the strategy has been set and then translated into objectives by the Department of Health it is passed to the Health Authorities. Their remit is to carry out an assessment of the health needs of their patient population.

As part of their role in meeting the needs of their local populations HAs carry out detailed and extended consultation exercises with representatives of local groups and with local GPs. As a result of this process, the Authorities publish an annual strategy document.

Provider units (Trusts) set their plan within the context of their purchaser's strategy. The Board of the Trust prepares corporate strategy documents for the organisation as a whole, while the individual component services, such as therapy services, build their individual business plans, which feed into the Trusts' overall plan.

In the NHS, service managers determine their own strategy within the context of the host organisation's goals and objectives, and budgetary constraints set by the purchaser, whilst at the same time managing within centrally determined budgets for their own particular service. For example, a therapy service within a Trust may be asked to develop a business plan which delivers the same number of episodes of care (activity) or an increased level, within the context of prescribed cost reductions.

Today, in practice, many therapy services operate service agreements between their individual service and their internal customers within the Trust and with any external customers, such as GPs. Clearly, this situation will alter depending on the organisational positioning of each therapy service. As such, it is relatively unusual for Health Authorities (purchasers) to concentrate on therapy service activity in isolation, but it is expected that this situation will change as PCGs emerge, and as purchasing becomes increasingly sophisticated in the future.

Strategic planning process

Using the overall corporate objectives and/or mission statement of the Health Authority and of the Trust itself, the business planning process for an individual service may involve the following seven steps:

- analysis of the service's external environment
- analysis of the service's internal environment
- selection of service objectives and goals
- development of service strategy
- preparation of operational plans
- development of implementation plan
- identification of feedback and control process.

Corporate objectives

Corporate objectives should provide the framework for each individual service's business plan. These objectives should include the Trust target population and population needs, where its services will be provided, the limits to service provision (e.g. service extension into the community) and the interface with other agencies. In addition, the objectives should indicate broad goals and values of the organisation.

Analysis of the external environment

The corporate objectives will help individual services to understand the direction that the host organisation wishes to pursue. Within this context managers of component services (therapies) will need to identify the threats and the opportunities relevant to their own service.

Opportunities

New opportunities should be identified and ranked in order of attractiveness and likelihood of success. Clearly, the ability of a service to exploit new opportunities successfully will depend on both its inherent strengths and the strengths of possible alternative service suppliers. However, strengths will change over time and so it is vital that this analysis is seen in the context of the service's ability to sustain its advantages over time.

Threats

Some developments in the health-care environment can be interpreted as potential threats. For example, a reduction in a service's budget will inevitably have implications for the resourcing of a service. Once identified, threats should be classified for the purposes of the business plan according to their degree of seriousness and probability of actually taking place.

Analysis of the internal environment: strengths and weaknesses

The analysis of strengths and weaknesses of a service needs to include marketing, financial, operational and managerial competencies. Judgement of each factor is commonly based on results of past performance and each service can rank the level of importance of each factor to the service as a whole on formulating its analysis of strengths.

In examining the results of the analysis, questions will be raised; for example, whether a service has the appropriate strength to exploit a new opportunity, or whether important weaknesses have been identified which will affect its reputation both within and outside the organisation as a whole.

Selecting service objectives

Once the service has examined the internal and external environment it is ready to identify its own separate goals and objectives. These will indicate what it wishes to achieve during the planning cycle. Typically, each service will agree several different objectives; it is helpful if these are arranged in order of importance. Each objective should be written in such a way as to be realistic (based on strengths and weaknesses), measurable (quantitative wherever possible), achievable within the timescale, and consistent and congruent with the mission statement and objectives of the organisation as a whole.

Developing strategy

Service goals give information about the direction in which a service wishes to travel, whilst strategy identifies how it will achieve its goals. In practice, strategy at therapy service level is commonly agreed through consultation and discussion with service members, although it is important to recognise that strategy is of itself dynamic in nature and, as such, will need to be revisited on a continuous basis.

Operational planning

Once the service has decided on its strategic ideas and goals, it must develop supporting operational programmes to implement its strategies.

For example, if a service has decided to become the leader in a particular new clinical speciality, it might include plans to:

- carry out research into the latest technological and clinical advances in the speciality
- design new service elements based on the research findings
- undertake a programme of training and development to enable staff to gain the requisite skills knowledge and competencies to operate the new scheme.

Implementation, feedback and control

Having carried out all elements of the business plan, it is vital that new work programmes be implemented soundly. Careful planning is required by managers to ensure that implementation proceeds according to agreed timescales, budgets and milestones.

Mechanisms are required to track the progress of implementation against agreed milestones over time and these mechanisms also need to identified as part of the business plan.

Tracking is essential, as it will allow managers to monitor progress and to make any necessary adjustments. The environment in which the organisation operates will continue to change; proper feedback and control mechanisms are essential to monitor progress against changes and against the agreed plan.

Contracting and commissioning

The impact of recent sets of reforms

The process by which funds are secured for the delivery of care services is probably the most complex aspect of NHS operations and one which has undergone the most numerous and profound changes in recent years. The process has been known variously as purchasing, contracting and commissioning, and is strongly linked to government policies.

The allocation of funds for care service provision in the UK was altered drastically with the introduction of the reforms in the late 1980s. Whilst NHS organisations had already entered into contractual arrangements with a number of external (including private) organisations for the supply of certain services (typically, catering and laundry services), no such arrangements existed between NHS organisations themselves. The 1980s' reforms changed this; purchasers' organisations (Health Authorities) and providers (NHS Trusts) contracted on an annual basis with each other, agreeing the services to be provided and the funding to support them.

These reforms brought with them huge organisational changes and also some criticism. Whereas the control of costs was welcome in the context of general financial constraint in the pubic sector, the resulting focus on financial measures rather than on clinical outcomes was unwelcome. The very short business planning cycle that accompanied annual contracting rounds was also felt to hamper the necessary longer term service development plans, including workforce plans, education and training commissions, which are so critical to NHS operations.

Commissioning and fundholding

During the early 1990s, at the same time as contracting arrangements were put in place between Trusts and Health Authorities, other forms of funding arrangements for care services developed in parallel. These concerned the primary care sector and, more specifically, GPs. Although their status as independent contractors never changed, certain GPs started to manage directly elements of their budgetary allocations. As usual for GPs, the allocations flowed via the Family Health Service Authorities (which later became subsumed into the Health Authorities); however, some GPs, especially those in quite large practices, were able to control directly an element of their funds and redeploy these under certain conditions as fundholders. Fundholders were able to reinvest savings made on the budgetary allocation that they controlled (typically through tighter control on prescribing) into new services for their patients. They could, for instance, recruit a physiotherapist to offer assessment and advice services to patients registered with them.

Over time, many variations on the fundholding system developed. These included:

- *multifunds*, where several fundholding GP practices combined and thus commanded control over larger funds, as each fundholding practice controlled an element of its budgetary allocation
- *total purchasing practices*, where practices controlled their entire budgetary allocation.

At the same time, the government published new White Papers on primary care provision and the concept of commissioning rather than fundholding was developed. Many GPs had resisted the introduction of fundholding on the grounds that it fostered the two-tier system, where patients who were registered with a fundholding GP potentially received more primary care services than those who were not. None the less, many of these GPs were keen to be involved more closely in the funding and organisation of primary care services and a number of GP commissioning pilot projects was started.

The likely shape of things to come

At the time of writing, the current government announced its plans for the organisation and funding of the NHS as part of the many changes introduced in a variety of White and Green Papers. The basic principle of GP commissioning was adopted, and the involvement of both GPs and community nurses in primary care service delivery, organisation and funding was announced via the development of PCGs. At their inception, the precise structure and remit of these PCGs was the object of much debate; PCGs are expected by the government and the NHS Executive to develop in scope over time. None the less, it can already be said that these new organisations (and later, PCTs) are likely to gain increasing importance over Health Authorities in the allocation of funds and the organisation of primary care services. They will also be expected to incorporate a measure of outcome in their commissioning activities. As the new commissioning arrangements emerge, their link to related care sector organisations' funding arrangements (e.g. SSDs in Local Authorities) will also be reviewed. This will ensure that public moneys are deployed to the maximum benefit of the population at large.

The changes in contracting and commissioning processes in the NHS over the years clearly illustrate that the way in which care services are funded heavily influences how they are organised. Finally, changes in funding flows also influence the relative powerbase of different stakeholders such as GPs, NHS Trusts and Health Authorities.

Therapy services: organisation in provider units

At a macro level, the key issues influencing therapy services in today's health-care business include the introduction and increasing sophistication of an internal health market, together with a gradual shift in emphasis of service provision from secondary to primary and community care. At a micro level, therapists have found themselves in new, and sometimes frequently changed, organisational structures; therefore, they now face a very different working environment to that of their colleagues in the mid-1990s.

Therapists, like most other professional groups in the NHS, have faced several reorganisations in the recent past, along with revised working policies and practices following each reorganisation. As a result, many structures and management arrangements have not been in place for long enough to be fully evaluated.

Trusts have a range of set-ups for the organisation of Professions Allied to Medicine (PAMs) and therapy services: full devolution to localities and clinical directorates, centrally managed, therapy directorates or agencies. There is no strong evidence to suggest that the choice of structure adopted is grounded in research; reasons for setting up devolved structures are often quoted as more cost effective or patient focused. This is an important point as there is a current trend for devolving centralised therapy services to localities and directorates. Many therapists find this threatening to their professional identity and ways of working.

Models of therapy services

A recent research report, 'Providing Therapists Expertise in the New NHS: Developing a Strategic Framework for Good Patient Care' (*Practices made Perfect*, Department of Health, 1997) examined different organisational structures that were prevalent in English Trusts. It found that there were four general models:

- therapy services managed as individual groups, headed by a senior member of that profession
- different therapy services managed as a combined professional group, headed by a person who may have a therapy professional background
- some parts of the services devolved to other organisational groupings, such as locality resource groups, or clinical directorates
- therapy services provided by external therapy service providers, such as from the private sector, or by staff from other NHS Trusts.

In between these arrangements, there is a wide variety of models. More recently, the growth of devolved structures has resulted in the emergence of other models; for example, models that comprise groups of therapists from different employing Trusts brought together and managed on an agency basis for their customers' benefit. It is not difficult to extrapolate from such a model similar structures which, managed effectively, could appeal to purchasing PCGs. Further details of various therapy organisational structures and their advantages and disadvantages are described in Chapter 3.

Clearly, the business planning process will vary according to the model of therapy service within a particular provider organisation. For example, therapists working within a clinical directorate structure may be involved in business planning in a multidisciplinary setting across the directorate as a whole, rather than simply in a uniprofessional dimension.

Therapy services and quality

The report 'Providing Therapists Expertise in the New NHS: Developing a Strategic Framework for Good Patient Care' (*Practices made Perfect*, Department of Health, 1997) also identified three main factors for delivering good patient care: efficacious practice, effective management and efficient service delivery. The report suggests that each individual service agree acceptable weightings for the factors with their staff, but suggested weightings could be:

- efficacious practice: 40%
- effective management: 30%
- efficient delivery: 30%.

The current government's drive to place an increased emphasis on quality in judging an individual Trust's performance focuses on the issues of clinical effectiveness and service evaluation.

To date, assessments of Trust performance and, within this, service evaluation have used 'hard' measures, such as activity (episodes of care), financial targets, waiting times and waiting list results. In the future, we can expect to see closer matching of these measures with indicators that inform both the purchasers and the public about the Trusts' clinical performance. Such a framework may use quality standards developed by professional bodies as a starting point; the ultimate aim is for each service to demonstrate that the practice of its clinical staff is based on sound research which demonstrates effective practice.

Such an approach poses challenges to therapy professions, where research into effectiveness for clinical procedures has been somewhat lacking in the past. Similarly, in terms of service evaluation, we may expect criteria to involve quality measures, set within the context of a national framework. The NICE and CHI are expected to contribute to the development of national frameworks for clinicians to use on a regular and frequent basis.

Beneath this, of course, is the need for every service to have robust and sound processes and systems for recording, collecting, analysing and reporting accurate and timely information about procedures used by clinicians in the variety of clinical settings in which they operate.

Other agencies

There are several important agencies outside the NHS, in addition to patients themselves and their carers, which relate to therapy services. They include:

- therapy user groups: Community Health Councils, special interest groups
- voluntary and independent sector organisations, Local Authorities (SSDs and LEAs)
- professional bodies
- research organisations.

The current government has placed significant emphasis on services' ability to deliver more closely integrated care by lessening the boundaries between the above organisations and the NHS; thus, in the future, we can expect increased efforts by major public sector bodies involved in health and social care to work more closely together on a practical level. Changes resulting from more seamless care may result in improved care delivery for patients and their carers, and reduce duplication of clinicians' work on a daily, practical basis on the part of clinicians.

Summary

This chapter has described how NHS funds are dispersed to the service through the Department of Health and NHS Executive to the remaining NHS bodies, and how the NHS reforms of the late 1980s introduced the concept of the internal market and separate health-care purchasers and providers. The latest reforms include the abolition of the internal market and the introduction of clinical governance. Over time, HAs will relinquish their commissioning activities to PCGs/PCTs, who will also manage their cash allocations for all health services within a unified health budget.

Our Healthier Nation represents a first step towards a national health promotion strategy and *A National Framework for Assessing Performance* proposes a framework against which NHS services are to be assessed in the future. Corporate and business planning in the NHS is driven by the strategy for the service, set out by the Secretary of State for Health; Health Authorities and Trusts work towards the implementation of this strategy through their corporate and business plans. PCGs/PCTs are likely to gain an increasingly important role in the future provision of health care.

In future, service providers may be expected to provide both 'hard' and 'soft' information as an indicator of their performance. The central drive to encourage a reduction in the boundaries between different care organisations may continue to promote the concept of further integration of therapy service provision.

Chapter 3
The Professions Allied to Medicine

Introduction

The health-care workforce can be divided into two main groups of staff: medical and non-medical. The nursing profession is the largest of the non-medical professional groups, representing approximately half of the total health service workforce. There are approximately 500,000 registered general nurses in the UK (UKCC, personal communication, 1998). The Professions Allied to Medicine (PAMs) are incorporated within this non-medical group and comprise approximately 10% of the workforce (Ham, 1991). With the total number of registered PAMs in the UK close to 100,000 (Council for the Professions Supplementary to Medicine, 1998), they represent a significant component of the overall health-care workforce.

To help the reader to understand some of the issues faced by the PAMs in the current and future health-care environment, this chapter describes the development of PAMs and how this relates to the current organisation of therapy services. In addition to considering the advantages and disadvantages of different organisational structures, the chapter considers how these organisational changes have impacted on the therapy professions and likely influences for the future. For the latter, particular attention is paid to the implications for career structures.

Defining the Professions Allied to Medicine

The term Professions Allied to Medicine was originally used to refer to those professions which were covered by the Professions Supplementary to Medicine (PSM) Act 1960 and regulated by the Council for the Professions Supplementary to Medicine. These professions currently include:

- physiotherapists
- occupational therapists
- radiographers (diagnostic and therapeutic)
- podiatrists and chiropodists
- orthoptists
- medical laboratory scientific officers
- dietitians
- art and drama therapists.

The total number of registered PAMs in the UK is close to 100,000 (Council for the Professions Supplementary to Medicine, 1998). Physiotherapy is the largest of these groups, with nearly 29,000 registered members, while art and drama therapists form the smallest group with fewer than 100 members.

There are several other professions with similarities to the above which are not strictly included in this definition of PAMs because they are not currently covered by the PSM Act. These professional groups include speech and language therapists, clinical psychologists and pharmacists. In the future, it is likely that ambulance paramedics, prosthetists and orthotists, audiologists, and speech and language therapists will join the PAMs group and be encompassed within the Act.

It is becoming increasingly common to consider all professionals under an umbrella term of health-care professions. Some recent research has considered these as PAMs (Standring, 1997; NHS Executive, 1998). However, there remains a plethora of terms used to describe more clearly this group of professions: diagnostic and therapy professions, clinical support services, therapy services or rehabilitation services. These terms attempt to embrace all non-medical professionals dealing with a similar patient interface, irrespective of whether or not their professional activity is regulated by the PSM Act 1960.

This chapter considers issues pertinent to many of the professions in any of the above definitions, but which are of particular relevance to the therapy professions.

Development of the Professions Allied to Medicine

Many of the PAMs have a long history and have experienced considerable professional growth, both in numbers and in stature, during the life of the National Health Service (NHS). During the 1980s and 1990s many of them underwent further significant growth and development. There have been two major influences on the development of these professions.

Firstly, there has been extensive development of preregistration education frameworks as the professions moved from postregistration diplomat status to all graduate professions. The reasons behind the shift to all graduate development at preregistration level were:

- the need for increased academic rigour
- the need for evidence-based practice and demonstrable clinical effectiveness requiring professionals with evaluative and research skills
- improved professional status
- the striving for increased professional autonomy.

Although some of these PAMs had professional autonomy prior to the 1980s, others did not and the exact nature of their work was normally determined by medical practitioners. Graduate status brought the majority of these professions greater autonomy although some, such as occupational therapists, still require medical referral. This autonomy has necessitated that the professions become increasingly active in research and evaluative of their clinical practice.

The second major change has been the growth in numbers of professionals and professional groups. For example, cumulative growth rates for occupational therapy and physiotherapy have been predicted at 17 and 32%, respectively, for the period 1993–1998 (EL(95)96, 1996). Despite this considerable growth, the demand for therapy services still outstrips supply. This demand is likely to increase further as awareness of the scope for using therapists to deliver patient care in today's health-care environment is recognised.

More recently, there has been increased emphasis on developing the professional role of PAMs, particularly related to extending the scope of clinical practice (e.g. radiographers developing skills in radiology; physiotherapists using joint injection). There is much debate about this issue. Increasingly, these professionals are becoming the first contact with the NHS in the secondary care setting, rather than a medical consultant.

Current organisation of therapy services

The majority of therapy services is currently provided by NHS provider units, i.e. Acute Trusts, Community Trusts and Specialist Trusts. Each Trust operates under an independent management structure, employing its own staff, including nursing and other support staff. However, the arrangements in place for the management of therapy staff are variable. Community Trusts and Specialist Trusts may purchase their therapy services from the therapy service of an Acute Trust or the reverse may apply. When this occurs, therapy service staff working in the Trust buying in the service are managed via the Trust providing the service. The providing and purchasing Trusts have a service agreement, which acts as a contract regarding the services provided and received. In addition to NHS provider units providing therapy services, independent therapy practitioners may be able to tender for therapy service contracts.

The management of staff working in therapy services has changed considerably as a result of the NHS reforms introduced in the early 1990s. Prior to 1989 a manager of the same professional background always managed staff of a particular profession. This arrangement now rarely exists: it is common practice for a single manager to be responsible for the management of a number of related professions (e.g. physiotherapists, occupational therapists, dieticians, and speech and language therapists may be managed by an occupational therapist). The manager is usually a member of one of the professions being managed, although this is not always the case.

Within each NHS Trust, services are frequently organised within a directorate structure. Directorates are usually led by a Clinical Director who is normally, although not always, a member of the medical profession. Directorates are commonly developed around the client base that they serve (e.g. medicine, surgery, the elderly). The way in which the therapy services are arranged and provided to these clinical areas is variable.

The following section details commonly utilised ways for organising therapy services within Trusts and highlights the advantages and disadvantages of each model.

Model 1

All therapy services are managed within a single directorate along with many other non-therapy services and delivered within a single setting (i.e. acute or community). For example, a Clinical Support Services directorate which holds service agreements with other directorates (see Fig. 3.1).

Advantages

- Maintains professional networks as channels of communication continue to exist freely within the professional groups
- better opportunities for in-house staff development
- immediate line management tends to be from similar discipline; therefore, greater understanding of professional need.

Disadvantages

- May not encourage multidisciplinary working because professional groups tend to remain unidisciplinary
- loss of professional identity as many other non-therapy professions managed within the same directorate.

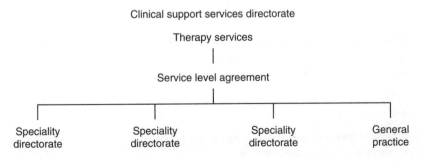

Fig. 3.1

Model 2

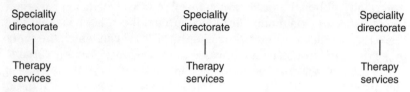

Fig. 3.2

Therapy services are organised within individual speciality directorates (i.e. each directorate employs its own therapy service staff rather than holding a service level agreement with another directorate) (see Fig. 3.2).

Advantages

- Very close liaison with staff of speciality directorate encourages strong speciality teamwork
- attractive to specialist staff
- potential benefits for the quality of service delivery as speciality directorate wholly focused on patient need
- professionals have better understanding of each others' roles and of integrated care.

Disadvantages

- Fragmentation of therapy services, especially smaller professional groups who may not be fully represented in each directorate
- probably no cover for sickness, holiday, etc.
- for therapists, possible lack of access to therapists in other specialisms for clinical advice
- professionals can feel isolated.

Model 3

In the Rehabilitation or Therapy directorate model, all therapy services are managed within one directorate; other non-therapy services are not managed within the directorate (see Fig. 3.3).

Advantages

- Reduces internal organisational boundaries
- strong rehabilitation focus
- therapy service staff have a very strong sense of identity

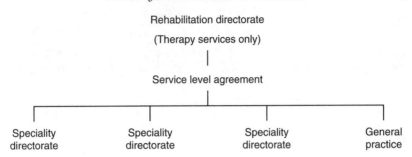

Fig. 3.3

- self-regulation
- excellent opportunities for the formation of interprofessional teams of therapists to develop strong integrated care for patients.

Disadvantages

- Specialities feel that they do not have ownership of staff and resources
- service planning and delivery is not focused on a speciality or disease
- can lead to the development of many small speciality 'therapy' teams.

Model 4

Therapy services operate independently of NHS Trusts (i.e. provided by the private sector) but hold individual contracts with Primary Care Groups (PCGs) (see Fig. 3.4).

Advantages

- Professional autonomy
- self-management and regulation.

Disadvantages

- Professional isolation
- limited opportunity for interprofessional working
- uniprofessional development very difficult to organise across wide geographical areas.

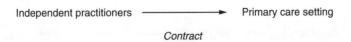

Fig. 3.4

Model 5

Therapy services work across the primary/secondary care boundary, following patient pathways. This type of service is likely to become more common in the future as confederations of professionals increasingly work across organisational boundaries.

Traditional model

See Fig. 3.5.

Future model

See Fig. 3.6.

Advantages

- Seamless care
- communication channels tend not to break down
- continuity of patient care provides high level of service efficiency
- reduces the number of professionals with whom each patient has to deal.

Disadvantages

- Sickness or holiday cover by staff who may be unfamiliar with caseload and clients.

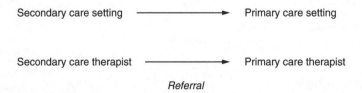

Fig. 3.5   Traditional model.

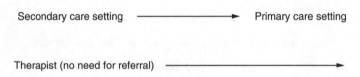

Fig. 3.6   Future model.

Development of current organisational structures

The ways in which services are currently organised exist for a number of reasons.

The health service manager of the early 1980s was probably more recognisable as having administrative rather than managerial duties. He or she was reactive rather than proactive (Harrison & Pollitt, 1994) and there was no formal accountability or quality framework of any kind for the services which were provided. *Working for Patients* (Department of Health, 1989b) was the main influence for fundamental change in the organisation of all health services; therapy services were not excluded from the changes which were to ensue.

The main components and implications of *Working for Patients* are given in Chapter 2. The reader is referred to Chapter 2 for the necessary background to the following section of this chapter. Of particular note, however, has been the increasing drive towards community-based services. Through Community Care policy (Department of Health, 1989a, 1993), Community NHS Trusts have become increasingly important in delivering care, although the more recent changes may see many of their services devolved to PCGs. Also of note was the development of health improvement targets to address major problem areas such as cardio-vascular disease, mental health, cancers and accidents (Department of Health, 1992). As key issues, both the development of community services and the health improvement targets attracted additional resources and, as a result, therapy services associated with them grew in size and stature.

Implications of current NHS organisation for the Professions Allied to Medicine

The internal market, created by the NHS reforms of the early 1990s, aimed to introduce competition into the health-care system, using this to drive improvements in cost effectiveness and efficiency and to improve quality. The strong emphasis on competition created barriers between hospital departments, Trusts and staff, who were reluctant to share information, expertise or resources, resulting in poor communication.

With the evolution of NHS Trusts as self-governing entities, therapy services became fragmented, a particular problem for the smaller professions. This impacted on the education and training of both students and junior staff and opportunities for collaborative working (Millar, 1998a). Joint development between therapy services and Health Authorities (NHS Executive, 1997a) was negligible, hindering service development and innovation.

Overview of career structures

The grading structures for PAMs are similar and generally follow those of the Whitley Council (PT 'A') terms and conditions of employment. Exceptions exist where local bargaining has resulted in Whitley arrangements being replaced by local contract terms. Further details of this are given in Chapter 7.

Over recent years, organisational structures have become flatter and, as a consequence, the career pathways for the therapy professions have become shorter (NHS Executive, 1998). Career advancement for PAMs can occur in three main areas:

- clinical
- managerial
- academia/research and development.

Each of these is considered in turn.

Clinical

With the exception of speech and language therapy, clinical grades for PAMs within the NHS fall into the following main categories:

- Junior/Basic grade
- Senior II
- Senior I
- Superintendent IV/Head IV/Chief IV
- clinical specialist/assistant.

Speech and language therapists have three main grades, with a range of salary spine points for Grades II and III. Occupational therapists working for Local Authority or Social Services have a grading structure similar to the NHS, although there are very few, if any, of the more junior grades.

Career progression in clinical grades normally takes a typical course. A newly qualified member of staff usually takes up a Junior/Basic grade position immediately upon qualification, where they are under the direct clinical supervision of a higher graded therapist. In some professions this position would be rotational (i.e. the staff member moves every 3 or 4 months around a series of different clinical specialities). After 1–2 years, the junior therapist normally progresses to a Senior II position, which carries more responsibility such as the management of other qualified or unqualified staff. At this grade the individual would tend to work without direct supervision. Posts at this level may be:

- static (the therapist remains in one clinical locality or speciality)

- rotational (the therapist continues to rotate among various specialities but spends longer periods in each, maybe 6–12 months)
- specialist rotation (the therapist rotates across several related clinical settings or specialisms).

After at least a further 2 years' experience, further clinical career progression is to Senior I grade. At this grade the therapist may work single-handedly and is expected to be undertaking highly skilled and specialised work. Senior I positions are considered to be the career grade for most of the therapy professions and an individual will normally attain this level after about 6–7 years' continual employment in their profession.

Recently, there has been moves to progress further the career grades at this level through the development of specialist practitioner positions. There is some inconsistency in the way that these posts have developed. In some units they have been awarded to individuals who demonstrate high levels of specialist skill, while in others they have been used to reward therapists involved in service development or evaluating the evidence base for therapy services. At the time of writing, there is no recognised Whitley Council salary for these specialist posts. The most recent recommendations from the Pay Review Body for PAMs (Pay Review Body, 1998) endorse the use of three discretionary increments which may be used for the most senior clinicians (those at the top of Senior II, Senior I, Superintendent IV/Head IV/Chief IV, Superintendent III/Head III/Chief III). In addition, the Pay Review Body recommended that the PT 'A' Whitley Council 'agree criteria for the operation of the system'. These criteria have recently been developed and will soon become operational. There continues to be increasing clinical opportunities for some therapists outside the NHS. For example, physiotherapists may hold clinical posts within occupational health services of large commercial companies, dietitians may work for firms that make special food products and any PAM may work in other health-related industries such as pharmaceuticals.

Managerial

Grades above Senior I (or equivalent) accrue a greater degree of management responsibility and tend to require Superintendent/Head/Chief grading. Career progression in the management grades tends to be upwards through Grades III to I, as shown:

- Superintendent III/Head III/Chief III
- Superintendent II/Head II/Chief II
- Superintendent I/Head I/Chief I.

In general, a therapist working at Superintendent I/Head I/Chief I level may still undertake some clinical work, but they are likely to have significant managerial responsibility. Where this responsibility spans more than one profession they are often referred to as therapy service managers.

Whilst the professional career structure in the managerial field is as indicated above, other career opportunities exist for therapists within the wider arena of health service management. However, in practice, relatively few therapists choose to move out of their professional arena.

Academia/research and development

A move into academia generally involves moving from the NHS into the higher education sector, although there remain one or two exceptions to this model. Research and development opportunities are becoming increasingly common in the NHS and tend to be linked to Senior clinical positions. An increasingly common opportunity is that of combined lecturer/practitioner appointments which foster links between academic and clinical settings.

The future

In late 1997 the government released its 10-year plan for the NHS. *The New NHS: Modern–Dependable* (Department of Health, 1997) initiates a further period of significant change for the NHS. The plan has three key themes of particular importance to PAMs.

Firstly, there is a continued drive to move health services into primary care. The formation of PCGs and then Primary Care Trusts (PCTs) will facilitate this. The second theme promotes high-quality, evidence-based health care, which will be monitored via a National Performance Framework. A National Institute for Clinical Excellence (NICE) will determine at a national level the best clinical practice based on available evidence. This will dictate the nature of services delivered. The third theme addresses the issue of equality of access to high-quality services.

The implications of these themes and other issues in the new NHS for PAMs are significant and many. There will be a continued move towards therapy services being delivered in the primary care or community setting. At the time of writing, it remains unclear how therapy services will be impacted by the development of PCGs. Despite support for consultation with PAMs, there is currently some fear that they will be excluded from dialogue during the early development period.

Longer term contracts, probably 3–5 years (EL(97)39, 1997), will give greater job security to staff and improve morale, which has suffered over recent years as a consequence of increased vulnerability. There is a strong commitment to working in partnership (Millar, 1998b) which should facilitate working between Trusts, Health Authorities, Local Authorities and voluntary agencies. In particular, local links with Social Services and Education Authorities will be targeted (Millar, 1998a) to help to reduce inappropriate medical referral, enhance opportunities for early interventions and improve communication.

Through participation in clinical governance, therapy services will be more accountable for service quality, both clinical and operational. There will be real emphasis on evidence-based practice, research and clinical audit.

Changes to the PSM Act 1960 will almost certainly recommend mandatory continuing professional development (CPD) for professional reregistration. This is likely to be organised as self-regulation via professional bodies. Most professional groups have a CPD strategy and many recommend the use of professional portfolios to record professional development.

In considering the future, one cannot ignore the ageing population. The number of people over the age of 85 years has doubled since 1981 and will double again by 2050 (Audit Commission, 1997). It has been suggested that 40% of acute admissions in the over-75 age group can be avoided (Audit Commission, 1997). One of the factors contributing to these hospital admissions is the lack of sufficient community rehabilitation services. In addition, early discharge from hospital can be facilitated by improved access to community-based rehabilitation (Audit Commission, 1997). Thus, it is likely that more therapy services will be focused on preventing admissions to and facilitating discharge from hospital. Programmes such as START (short-term assessment and rehabilitation teams) and outreach services (Chadda, 1998) can help to achieve this goal.

Demand for therapy services will continue to grow and is always likely to be much greater than supply. Serious consideration will need to be made to the future configuration and skill mix of therapy services if this demand is going to be met.

The future delivery of therapy services is likely to involve greater teamwork across organisational and agency boundaries. The use of integrated care pathways and outreach/inreach services, centred on individual client groups (Riley, 1998), is probable: current care pathways are mainly used in the acute setting and are not extensively used in the UK (Riley, 1998).

Greater emphasis on health promotion and health education will be evident in striving to achieve health improvement targets (Department of Health, 1998). There will be continued emphasis on multiprofessional working, education and training, at both preregistration and postregistration levels (SCOPME, 1997). Those employed within therapy services may well become involved in the telephone advice services set to be in place by the year 2000.

One further point worthy of consideration relates to service delivery, in that restriction to the traditional working hours of PAMs staff must be called into question. Services that are available from Monday to Friday, 8.30 a.m. to 4.30 p.m. cannot be considered accessible to service users who are not hospital patients. This also applies to services provided at weekends and on bank holidays. Therapists must take a long, hard look at the way in which services are delivered: current working patterns must change if the full benefit of therapy services is to be realised. Current service delivery hours do not meet or respect patients' needs.

There are many challenges ahead. The only certainty is that there will be ongoing change to which the therapy services must respond. Therapy service deliverers have an enormous wealth of skill, knowledge, attitude and experience that can bear considerable fruit to the NHS of the future. Therapy services must be innovative and rise to this challenge.

Conclusion

There is a central and growing role for therapists in patient management in all areas of the NHS. The services that they provide 'are an integral part of the National Health Service and provide an important and valuable service to patients' (Langlands, 1997). The NHS will continue to change since 'change and transition are more typical of contemporary life than equilibrium and status quo' (Owen, 1996, cited by Harden, 1998). There are many excellent and innovative models for delivering rehabilitation services (NHS Executive, 1997b). In the future, therapists will have to continue to remain flexible in their approach to the delivery of care. Only then will they have any chance of meeting the constantly increasing and changing demand for their services.

References

Audit Commission (1997) *The Coming of Age: Improving Services for Older People*. Audit Commission, London.
Chadda, D. (1998) Budding relationship. *Health Service Journal* 26 March, 10–11.
Council for Professions Supplementary to Medicine (1998) Press release from Physiotherapists Board Meeting, 27 September.
Department of Health (1989a) *Caring for People: Community Care in the Next Decade and Beyond*. HMSO, London.
Department of Health (1989b) *Working for Patients*. HMSO, London.
Department of Health (1992) *Health of the Nation*. HMSO, London.
Department of Health (1993) *Community Care in the Next Decade and Beyond*. HMSO, London.
Department of Health (1997) *The New NHS: Modern–Dependable*. HMSO, London.
Department of Health (1998) *Our Healthier Nation*. HMSO, London.
EL(97)39 (1997) *NHS Priorities and Planning Guidance 1998/1999*. NHS Executive, Leeds.

Ham, C. (1991) *The New National Health Service*. Radcliffe Medical Press, Oxford.

Harden, R. (1998) Editorial: Change – building windmills not walls. *Medical Teacher* **20**(3), 189–91.

Harrison, S. & Pollitt, C. (1994) *Controlling Health Professionals: The Future Work and Organisation in the NHS*. Open University Press, Buckingham.

Langlands, A. (1997) *Foreword to Providing Therapists' Expertise in the New NHS: Developing a Strategic Framework for Good Patient Care*. NHS Executive, Leeds.

Millar, B. (1998a) This time it's real. *Health Service Journal* 26 March, 14.

Millar, B. (1998b) Local colour. *Health Service Journal* 2 April, 15.

NHS Executive (1997a) *Providing Therapists' Expertise in the New NHS: Developing a Strategic Framework for Good Patient Care*. NHS Executive, Leeds.

NHS Executive (1997b) *Rehabilitation – A Guide*. NHS Executive, Leeds.

NHS Executive (1998) *NHS Career Development Initiative for the Professions Allied to Medicine*. NHS Executive, Leeds.

Pay Review Body (1998) Review body for nursing staff, midwives, health visitors and professions allied to medicine: Fifteenth Report on Professions Allied to Medicine 1998 – Main Findings and Recommendations. Department of Health, London.

Riley, K. (1998) Paving the way. *Health Service Journal* 26 March, 30–1.

SCOPME (1997) Multiprofessional working and learning: sharing the educational challenge (SCOPME Working Paper).

Standring, J. (1997) The NHS Career Development Initiative for the Professions Allied to Medicine (NHS Executive – North West Regional Report). NHS Executive North West Regional Office.

Further reading

Flynn, R., Williams, G. & Pickard, S. (1996) *Markets and Networks: Contracting in Community Health Services*. Open University Press, Buckingham.

Glynn, J.J. & Perkins, D.A. (Eds) (1995) *Managing Health Care: Challenges for the '90s*. W.B. Saunders, London.

Holliday, I. (1995) *The NHS Transformed*. Baseline, Manchester.

Klein, R. (1992) *The Politics of the NHS*. Longman, London.

Chapter 4
Getting Started in a Job

Introduction

Starting a first job is recognised as one of the transition points in life and can be an awesome experience, as can changing jobs. In many ways those who embark on professional training have already made decisions regarding the general direction of their career path; in other words, they have chosen to work in a particular professional area. Both this, and practical training undertaken within the undergraduate curriculum, mean that new Professions Allied to Medicine (PAMs) already have some experience and knowledge of the type of environment they can expect to work in. This chapter aims to raise awareness about other issues which PAMs can expect employers to consider when recruiting staff and employers' expectations of employees. It initially considers the stages of a career, followed by details of the recruitment and induction processes.

Starting a career

Ball (1995) describes four useful stages for entering a career.

Designer stage

Most PAMs will have consciously or unconsciously been through this stage before embarking on their course of study. At this stage, through looking at your own skills, attributes and interests as well as investigating your own work values, you would have developed certain conclusions about the content or style of your preferred career. Most jobs centre around working with people, data or things.

Explorer stage

At this stage, you look at all available options. Therapists, fortunately, have a wide variety of openings available to them, some of which are described in Chapter 10. For therapists, it is at this point that you must consider the type and breadth of experience offered by a particular employing organisation as well as identify where you will feel most able to become an effective member of a team or department (e.g. whether you enjoy being part of a large organisation, such as a teaching hospital, or would prefer a smaller environment, such as a community-based team).

Researcher stage

This stage involves getting to know the different organisations that have vacancies which match your interests and aspirations – this could be crucial to how your career progresses in the future. Most organisations now have information packs that are sent to prospective employees. Studying these carefully should give some feel of the organisation's philosophy and their commitment to staff. The nationally recognised 'Investors in People' award demonstrates standards in staff support, training and development, and is a good indicator of an organisation's standing. The way in which jobs are advertised also indicates an organisation's attitude: some advertisements offer informal visits or chats. Such opportunities will provide further information about both the organisation and the job and, as such, pursuance of these is encouraged.

Promoter stage

Having decided that an organisation is right for you, you need to make potential employers see that you are right for them and the job on offer. Thus, this stage is about self-marketing: it is important to get yourself recognised. This can be done by attendance at open days or talking to people whom you wish to influence. When making a formal application, construct a good curriculum vitae (CV), which demonstrates written skills. The CV should indicate your range of skills, levels of experience and the degree to which you are willing to have a flexible approach to your work.

For some, the transition from student life to the reality of working life means initial feelings of insecurity and lack of confidence owing to inexperience or concerns regarding acceptance by others. Whether leaving university and entering the labour market or moving from one organisation to another, some forethought is required about both yourself and your own needs, as well as those of your prospective employer. Understanding the process of recruitment may aid in your successful appointment to the desired post.

The recruitment process

Recruitment can be is defined as *finding a suitable employee for an employer.* This may sound simple and straightforward but incorporates a complex chain of events and close integration of several systems to achieve this aim. The consequences of being unsuccessful can be far reaching and costly. Most organisations undertake the recruitment process internally, but some now ask recruitment agencies to assist them in the procedure.

Clarifying the job

Before any vacant position is advertised, the relevant manager or supervisor will have made a series of decisions about the job and its requirements. Firstly, they will have determined the job role by undertaking a job analysis. This process systematically examines a job as a vacancy arises, recognising that jobs change over time. A vacancy creates a good opportunity to undertake such a review. Job analysis includes looking at the tasks to be performed, the responsibilities of the post holder, how the job relates to others and its requirements in terms of skills, knowledge and attributes, including qualifications and experience. An exit interview with the outgoing post holder is often part of this process.

The importance of this process must be understood, particularly if you are interested in an internal vacancy, especially for promotion. In such circumstances, it is worth discussing this with the manager responsible for advertising the job prior to submitting a job application. The job analysis process may mean that the vacant post has changed: the expectations of a new post holder may be different from the role performed by former colleagues.

All jobs require a job description. Although job descriptions are expected to describe a job in precise terms, they cannot possibly identify every single aspect of what a post holder is required to do. Normally, a job description gives a statement of the overall purpose of the job, where the post holder will fit into the organisation (including lines of accountability), as well as details of duties and responsibilities. In the past, most therapy jobs within the National Health Service (NHS) were governed by the Whitely Council PT 'A' terms and conditions of service. As NHS Trusts are individual employers, some have their own terms and conditions of service, and any differences in these from PT 'A' may be reflected in job descriptions (e.g. levels of responsibility; lines of accountability). There is no requirement for employers within the private or voluntary sector to adhere to any national guidance on the way in which a job is defined. This is worth remembering if considering posts within several organisations, so that necessary comparisons can be made; studying the job description should help you to be clear of the expectations of each post.

In addition to a job description, managers are advised to devise a person specification for the post. This outlines the personal characteristics and attributes desirable of the job holder. It will also describe minimum standards of qualification, experience, attainments and the physical requirements of the job. Person specifications should help you to decide your own suitability for the post on offer. The person specification is normally distributed with a job application form and job description; if these are not supplied, you should ask for them.

By studying these documents in detail, you can ascertain the criteria used by managers to shortlist potential applicants for the next stage in the recruitment process. These criteria will also be used for assessment at interview. By understanding these criteria, you will be able to complete the application form in a way which links your skills, attributes and experience to the requirements of the post. An informal visit prior to the closing date for job application may also help determine the most important criteria. Failing this, the only influence that a manager has on determining your suitability as a potential post holder is the information given on your application form. If the latter does not identify how you fit the requirements of the job, it is unlikely that you will be offered an interview or a further assessment.

Many job descriptions and person specification will use a variety of terms or phrases, the definitions of which may not be clear to new PAMs. The following paragraphs list some of these terms and describe what they mean to managers.

Fitness for purpose, fitness for practice

From the above, it is clear that managers go through several processes to recruit the right person to a job. Managers are interested in fitness for purpose when appointing staff to particular posts.

By attaining a degree, newly qualified PAMs or therapists will have satisfied their higher education institution or training school that they are fit for award by achieving the specified level of educational standards required for award. Several of the PAMs undergraduate courses are jointly validated by the relevant, individual professional body and the CPSM; qualification also ensures fitness to practice. This means that new graduates are able to practise safely in normal clinical situations and are state registered. This, however, does not mean that any newly qualified therapist or PAM is fit to fill any junior post. Despite being fit for award and fit for practice, you may not meet the requirements for a particular junior post (i.e. not fit for purpose). This may be because you may not have the specific competencies, skills, experience or personal attributes required for the job.

Competencies

Competencies are the core skills required to perform effectively at a given

grade or level and should create expectations which are mutually understood by both employer and employee. A clear set of competencies for
a given post provides a clear focus for appraisal and easy identification
of employee training or development needs. For example, in physiotherapy and occupational therapy (OT) some national work has been
undertaken in developing standards for first-post competencies covering
the first 2-year period post-qualification (North West Regional Health
Authority, 1992). These should be available in physiotherapy or OT training schools or NHS therapy departments and may help to monitor progress.

For those aiming to develop their career through promotion, competencies are equally important. You will already have experience of work
which has developed skills, knowledge and attitudes in your chosen profession. In addition to practical experience of work, you will have been
influenced by the working environment.

Competencies are usually considered under three main headings:
knowledge, skills and attitudes. Each of these is defined as follows.

- *Knowledge* is what you know. This may be knowledge related to a particular profession as well as more general knowledge.
- *Skills* are what you are able to do. They describe the capabilities of
  an individual to perform certain tasks. This may involve their ability
  to apply knowledge. Skills can be manual, technical or managerial.
  In today's labour market, transferable skills (e.g. communication, team
  working) are becoming increasingly important.
- *Attitudes* determine how a job or situation is approached and are
  based on an individual's values and beliefs. These can change over
  time and are influenced by previous experience. Rarely is the importance of an appropriate attitude to work openly acknowledged. Yet
  it is often the display of an inappropriate attitude at work which
  creates difficult problems. Issues around this are explored further in
  Chapter 5. It is common for newly qualified PAMs, with no or limited
  previous working experience, to have an attitude based on idealism;
  only after entering the workplace is this tempered with realism. Attitudes are becoming more important in today's working environment.
  The ability to have a flexible attitude and openness to change is now
  felt, by most managers, to be crucial. The changes outlined in the
  White Paper *The New NHS: Modern–Dependable* (Department of
  Health, 1997), which emphasise interdisciplinary working and inter-
  agency partnerships, will mean changes in attitude for many older or
  experienced therapists. In the future, therapists' jobs will require
  greater emphasis on sharing knowledge and skills as well as undertaking roles that they may not traditionally see as their own.

As professionals, it is expected that PAMs keep up to date with their
knowledge and skills through professional practice and by attending relevant, postgraduate training.

Minimum expectations

Employers' expectations of their potential employees form the basis of the judgements that they make during recruitment. Whilst the qualification that therapists receive through attaining their degree may ensure their safety to practice, there remains a great deal of practical experience and learning to become a recognised, effective practitioner. As well as assessment and treatment skills, there are other, more general attainments that make an individual fit for purpose. Some examples of these are listed below.

- *Effective time management*: it is a reasonable expectation that any clinical practitioner is able to manage their time at work and thus to manage their own caseload of patients. This will mean time spent on dealing directly with patients but also ensuring that clinical records and correspondence are updated within appropriate time frames (e.g. it is generally accepted that records of clinical interventions are written up within 12 hours of the intervention). Other demands on time include attending meetings, case conferences or training sessions. Therapists are also expected to prioritise work, especially their patient caseload. Many newly qualified therapists find time management difficult, and may also struggle to prioritise their caseload appropriately. Managers or supervisors will not find such difficulties surprising and will be able to offer considerable help. If informal advice is not sufficient, then more formal training can normally be arranged and is sometimes readily available through organisations' existing training schemes.
- *Research awareness*: in today's working environment, there is an expectation that clinicians be research aware and can reflect on both their own and others' clinical practice. This means being willing and able to stand back and evaluate their own clinical interventions, particularly in relation to published evidence and recognised good clinical practice. As the therapy professions progress, they will achieve greater success in and more opportunities to undertake their own research.
- *Professional accountability*: individual professions have their own code of ethics or conduct, mainly developed by professional bodies. These address the accountability issues associated with therapists' work with patients and colleagues. Further information on these is given in Chapters 3 and 9.
- *Effective communication*: communication is a major part of therapists' work. Well-developed verbal communication skills allow therapists to interview patients and carers effectively and communicate with a wide range of colleagues in various settings. Written communication abilities are also important. Accurate and thorough entries in patient records are as important as practical interventions, as

patients may rely on such recorded evidence in the future. As autonomous practitioners, therapists must be able to defend their actions should there be a litigation claim which involves their intervention or patient. Attention must also be paid to organisational policies and procedures.

- *Teamwork and roles*: therapists do not usually work in isolation, even if they are working alone. In most roles, they must develop relationships with a number of people and work in a variety of teams. There is thus an expectation that therapists are able to understand the role of others within a team, as well as their own, and know the limitations and boundaries of each. Teamwork is explored further in Chapter 5.

The recruitment interview

Full details of all aspects and permutations of interviewing and the interview process are beyond the scope and intention of this chapter; there are many other publications which deal with this issue (see the end of this chapter). This section will highlight a few key issues felt by the author to be of particular importance or relevance to PAMs.

Various people may be involved with the interview process and this will vary between different organisations and for different levels of job, depending on either the departmental or organisational recruitment policy. Usually, an interview panel will comprise a minimum of two people, although it may often comprise three or four. Whilst the larger number may appear more daunting, it has the advantages of increasing the reliability of judgements made by interviewers and in ensuring fair scoring.

Many organisations now use scoring systems to mark candidates at interview; the scoring criteria normally relate closely to the criteria set out in the job and person specifications.

Normally, an interview panel consists of those who were involved in the shortlisting process, with the possible addition of a representative of the personnel department to advise on the organisation's polices (e.g. relocation expenses). Typically, the immediate line manager associated with the post on offer and the manager of the department will be included in the interview panel. They are likely to be highly conversant with the job and know its requirements intimately. They should thus be able to answer any questions about the job. If the interviewers are not able to answer such questions adequately, it may be possible to ask to meet potential colleagues to explore the questions further with them. As well as the interviewers' deciding on the suitability of a candidate for the post, the candidate should feel confident and happy about accepting any post offered.

Some organisations expect candidates to give a presentation as well as undergo an interview, especially for senior or promotional posts. In such a situation, candidates must be prepared to respond to questions about the presentation as well as answer formal interview questions.

Other aspects of recruitment

Medical assessment

If a post is offered to a candidate after interview, it is normal for the job offer to be subject to satisfactory medical screening and references. Medical assessment is usually organised by the occupational health department of the organisation offering the job. Occasionally, some organisations will allow the occupational health department of a current employer to undertake a similar medical assessment.

Pre-employment health screening is usually undertaken by an occupational health nurse or doctor. It aims to identify the likelihood of risk to the employer from an existing health or medical problem. The process normally involves a health-screening questionnaire and, if deemed necessary, a physical examination. The process also ensures that staff are protected by relevant inoculations and that they are physically fit to undertake the requirements of the post. It is important that any medical problems are declared at this stage. For example, disciplinary action may result if an employee has difficulty with attendance at work as a result of a known medical problem that was not declared at the time of the pre-employment examination.

Legal issues

The process of recruitment is governed by a range of Employment Law legislation. The most significant of these to PAMs are summarised below.

- *The Sex Discrimination Act 1975* makes it unlawful to discriminate on grounds of sex in full- or part-time employment, training and other related matters. Discrimination means treating a person less favourably than another because of their sex. The Act also applies to discriminatory advertising and discriminating against a person owing to their marital status, in both prospective and existing employment.
- *The Race Relations Act 1976* makes it unlawful to discriminate on grounds of race during the recruitment process and the terms under which a job offer is made or not made. For existing employees, the Act makes racial discrimination unlawful where race is the basis on which employees are treated or managed differently in any way (e.g. how they are treated in promotion opportunities, training, disciplinary procedures).

- *The Disabled Persons (Employment) Act 1995* requires employers to treat disabled persons in the same way as non-disabled persons in all employment matters. Employers are also expected to make reasonable changes to premises, work layout and hours of work to accommodate the needs of a disabled employee. Under this Act, disablement includes sensory and mental deficits as well as physical problems. The Act also governs the provision of goods and services, including any type of therapy service. That is, the services provided to disabled people have to be the same as those services offered to non-disabled persons. Any resulting change in premises or service provision must comply with health and safety laws.
- *The Equal Pay Act 1970 [as amended by the Equal Pay (Amendment) Regulations 1983]* ensures equal treatment of men and women in the terms and condition of employment, including pay, for jobs that are broadly similar or have equal value. This applies to both full-time and part-time employees.
- *The Rehabilitation of Offenders Act 1974* allows an individual who has had a conviction and been rehabilitated to treat the conviction as if it had not occurred. The conviction is considered 'spent' if the individual has not, after a period of time, committed another serious offence. During recruitment the employer may not ask a prospective employee about any spent convictions. If the employer asks the individual about any convictions, the prospective employee is under no obligation to reveal spent convictions. The Act also makes it unlawful for employers to discriminate against an employee because of a spent conviction.

All organisations are required to monitor their performance against these laws. Job application packages from any prospective employer will usually contain a declaration form addressing the issues concerned.

Prospective employees who are expected to work with children will undergo further vetting prior to appointment. This vetting process, carried out via police services, ascertains past criminal records, with particular attention to offences against children.

The NHS has special regulations for certain health professional groups, whereby continued state registration with the appointed registration body is required as part of the employment contract. This covers most therapy professions, with the exception of speech and language therapy. Further details of state registration and its conditions are given in Chapters 3 and 9. Other legislative issues associated with the working environment are described in Chapter 6.

Induction to a new position

The process of induction helps new recruits to enter and deal with a new working environment. An induction programme is crucial, especially when an individual starts work in a new organisation. A good induction programme takes time and effort to arrange. Many organisations provide both corporate and departmental induction. This gives new employees an overview of the philosophy and overall direction of the organisation as well as details of departmental structures and procedures.

An induction programme should be offered on the first day with a new employer. A checklist is often provided to ensure that all relevant issues are addressed. An example of such a checklist is given in Fig. 4.1.

The induction process usually provides new recruits with the 'domestic' arrangements for the department in which they work, e.g. departmental layout and routine activities. There will be a range of departmental polices and procedures with which new employees must become familiar. In addition, details and expectations of aspects such as reporting of sickness or absence, application for leave, staff meeting times, appraisal systems, administration systems and record keeping should be provided.

The induction process provides information which is mandatory to all employees, including health and safety regulations (fire procedure, evacuation procedure, accident reporting, security arrangements). In some clinical areas, there may be special regulations (e.g. security for staff working in the community). Clinical staff can also expect induction to include resuscitation training or update, manual handling training and infection control procedures. As part of an organisation's risk-management strategy, many of these issues are subject to self-assessment and audit (see Chapter 6).

Normally, new recruits are given time to undertake other aspects of their induction as they feel necessary and at their own volition. This may include attending lectures, meeting new colleagues and undertaking specific training. The value of this time sometimes goes unrecognised; it is often the responsibility of the new recruit to use the time allocated for this purpose. The relevant line manager and other colleagues may give direction on how to use this time to best effect. Good induction saves a great deal of time in the following months.

Chapter 1 highlighted the importance of organisational culture and how this may influence how employees work. Understanding the culture of a new organisation will help new recruits to fit in more easily with the variety of teams within which they must work. This must be considered throughout the induction process and for some time afterwards.

Conclusion

Starting a first job or changing jobs can be an awesome experience. Whilst practical training undertaken within the undergraduate curriculum can

TOPIC	DATE	COMPLETED	SIGNED
'Housekeeping'			
Payment Method			
Leave Policy			
Sickness Reporting			
Lieu Time			
Health & Safety			
Occupational Health			
Fire Procedure			
Accident Reporting			
Security Badge			
Administration			
Secretarial Support			
Statistics / Data			
Record Keeping			
Photocopying			
Environment			
Department Tour			
Hospital Tour			
Hospital Map			
Unit Induction			
Professional Practice			
CPSM Certificate			
Information			
Induction Pack			
Health & Safety File			
Policy File			
Team Information			
Communication	Dates / Times / Venues Given		
Team Meetings			
Team Brief			
Staff Meetings			
Access to Manager	Name Tel Ext Bleep No		
Staff Side Representative	Name Tel Ext Bleep No		
Other			

Fig. 4.1   General induction checklist.

prepare new therapists for the clinical aspects of starting work, new PAMs may not be aware of other issues which may be of importance in their acquiring and settling into a job. This chapter has described issues which PAMs can expect employers to consider when recruiting staff and in the early stages of their working life. This should facilitate new PAMs in obtaining and getting to grips with their first job after qualification. It may also be of value to other therapists changing jobs or returning to the labour market after a career break.

References

Ball, B. (1995) *Managing your own Career.* British Psychological Society, Kogan Page, London.

Department of Health (1997) *The New NHS: Modern–Dependable.* HMSO, London.

NHS Executive North West Regional Health Authority (1992) *First Post Competencies.* Department of Health, London.

Further reading

Burt, S. (1993) *Preparing for Interviews.* Pitman Publishing, London.

Crabtree, S. (1991) *Moving Up – A Practical Guide to Career Advancement for Managers, Consultants and Professionals.* Kogan Page, London.

Higham, M. (1983) *Coping with Interviews.* New Opportunity Press, London.

McBride, P. (1993) *Excel at Interviews.* Hobsons CRAC, London.

Yate, M.J. (1992) *Great Answers to Tough Interview Questions – How to Get the Job You Want.* Kogan Page, London.

Chapter 5
Working With People

Jane is an occupational therapist working in a District General Hospital. She currently works on the stroke unit with two other occupational therapists. Every month there is a unit meeting for all clinical and managerial staff. The purpose of the meeting is to give staff the opportunity air their views, influence policy and share information. Jane is finding these meetings difficult. Over a cup of coffee, she complains that the consultant in charge doesn't seem to take anybody's views seriously. If anyone challenges a policy proposal or points out potential problems, they are dismissed as ill informed or negative. People seem to misinterpret, almost deliberately, what others are saying. For example, there was a discussion of a proposal on multidisciplinary notes which Jane had helped devise. People who had expressed support outside the meeting said nothing during it. The proposal was rejected, leaving Jane feeling exposed and isolated. Every now and then, however, things seem to work really well. She gave the example of a debate over the introduction of self-administration of drugs for selected patients. Although there wasn't unanimous support for the proposal, the issue was aired thoroughly. Everyone seemed happy they had had their say and been listened to, even if their preferred option was rejected in the end. Jane wondered why the same group could at function so well some times and so badly at others.

Introduction

Jane's problems with a team meeting are not atypical. The above scenario illustrates a complex combination of factors that influence personal and group behaviour, sometimes to good effect and sometimes not. Whatever your role or position, you can be sure that to achieve in your job, you must work with people. You will need to work with colleagues of the same and different professional groups; some will be in a line management relationship to you, while others will not. Some will be more senior than you or have more power than you. Some will be easy to work with, while others you will find difficult. Sometimes the relationships are individual and sometimes they are in teams.

This chapter aims to provide some insights and ideas about how to establish and sustain good working relationships in all of these situations. Firstly, the chapter introduces a model of understanding interpersonal relationships. Secondly, it explores particular issues presented by group or team working. Thirdly, it identifies constructive ways of handling difficult situations with individuals or in groups.

Working with individuals

Mistaken assumptions

Many problems at work can be clarified by realising that we often make inaccurate assumptions about other people. Two are very common.

- *Everyone shares the definition of the situation.* Most of us would accept that we tend to act upon what we perceive to be the reality of the situation. However, what may be the reality for one person may not be the reality for someone else. They may not agree about the problem, never mind the solution, because there is no agreement about the 'facts' of the situation. Even facts apparently beyond dispute, such as the state of the finances, are open to very different interpretations.

  In situations in everyday life, such as choosing friends, we gravitate towards those who seem to share our way of seeing the world and avoid those whose do not. However, we cannot pick and choose amongst work colleagues, so it is important to recognise the variety of differing definitions of the situation. It is not easy to accept that what may seem an irrational or distorted view to you, seems quite reasonable to those who hold it. However, once you have accepted this, there is a far better chance of understanding what is happening in meetings and you may be able to handle the situation more productively.
- *Everyone is working towards the same goals.* This is an equally dangerous assumption. The goals of both individuals and professional groups inevitably differ. For some, the goal may be to achieve personal career success; for others, the goal may be to protect their professional service from exploitation; and for yet others, the goal may be to balance the books. All may declare their commitment to an overarching goal of patient care, but this can often be obscured by more immediate concerns.

  Business plans, mission statements and objective setting may lead you to believe that all staff are – or should be – working towards the same goals across the organisation. There are, however, always individual and group agendas which may hamper realising such objectives. We tend to believe that people around us will almost naturally do whatever is necessary to achieve the 'agreed' organisational goals. Even when they do, there is a real chance that their actual motives have very little to do with the desire to meet those goals.

When working with people, there is always a need to appreciate and balance personal and organisational goals. Where these goals conflict, relationships will suffer.

Ego states

Eric Berne (1964) proposed that we all use a complex, shifting combination of distinctive conditions or states which he describes as ego states. Each ego state produces a very different sort of behaviour. Recognising which state we or a colleague occupy can be enormously helpful in understanding possible tensions or difficulties that may be encountered. There are three states.

- *The parent state* tends to display typical parental behaviour. It is concerned with authority, morality, judgement and guilt. Within this state Berne distinguishes two types of behaviour; that of the 'critical parent' and the 'nurturing parent'. Typically, someone operating in the critical parent state would communicate in a one-way fashion: telling, informing or instructing, leaving little room for response or dialogue. The nurturing parent, in contrast, would be characterised by protective behaviours: sympathetic and cosseting. Such behaviour implies dependency in others, assuming that they need looking after and are not yet ready to branch out on their own. Any kind of parental behaviour can, and often does, unwittingly stifle genuine learning and dialogue.
- *The child state* is characterised by accepting a dependency on others. It involves at least two different types of child-like behaviour. The first is the 'natural child', characterised by fun-loving, spontaneous and uninhibited behaviour. The second, the 'adapted child', is characterised by the more devious behaviour that we learn to use to obtain recognition or reward, such as flattery.
- *The adult state* is characterised by rationality and objectivity, dispassionate consideration of the facts. We operate in the adult state when we attempt to focus on reasons and seek the truth of a situation in a detached and an unemotional way.

Berne is a psychiatrist who believes that these states are fundamental to our sense of who we are and that we revert to them unconsciously in all kinds of situations. They are recognisable in our experience of family life, where we first learn them. Thus, at family celebrations we may find ourselves moving from an adult state with our partners or siblings, to a parental state with our children and to a child state when confronted by our own parents. Berne is suggesting that we also do this outside the family, even at work.

By recognising these three states, we can begin to understand the nature of the interactions between ourselves and those around us. Think about the last time your work was discussed with your line manager. In which state would you describe yourself? How did this affect your behaviour and, equally important, what reaction did your behaviour have upon your line manager? Often, in such an instance, there is a real danger of slipping into the child state in response to, or to elicit, parental behaviour from your manager.

In the example of Jane and the discussion over multidisciplinary patient notes, the way in which the problem was defined by individuals would have had a direct impact on their attitudes. What to one person may be a practical solution to too much paperwork, to another may be a threat to their established way of doing things, tied to their ideas about professional competence. Even if recognised as being in the best interests of the unit as a whole, the proposal might have been seen as requiring some individuals and groups to give up control of part of their 'patch'. Their personal goals were different from those of the organisation as a whole.

Berne's framework might suggest that the consultant tended to display a parental ego state, refusing to take the contribution of other staff seriously. This may have produced a number of reactions. The temptation to respond to the parent with the child ego state would have been considerable. Since this would complement the state adopted by the doctor, this would be comfortable for both parties. However, tension might have arisen if some staff refused to respond in the child state but adopted the adult state, expecting to be treated as equal partners in a frank discussion of the problem. Then the doctor would either have adopt a similar adult role himself or try to put them down in an attempt to restore his (parental) authority. Ideally, the consultant could have stopped trying to impose his reality on everybody else and negotiated with others' perceptions. This should remove the implied invitation to others to adopt the child ego and enable an adult/adult interaction. This case implies that this was achieved at another meeting when self-prescribing was discussed.

Working in teams

We do not always work in one-to-one situations. Often, we find ourselves working in teams of one sort or another. It is likely that through your career you will belong to a range of teams, sometimes simultaneously. There will be your team of colleagues from the same profession, the multidisciplinary team in your specialist field and other project teams that you join on a more temporary basis. It is often in teams that we get things done. What applies to individuals also applies to teams. The dangers lie in assuming that everyone shares the same definition of the situation and has common goals, and in adopting inappropriate ego states, but interactions in teams involve consideration of different kinds of behaviour.

The individual in the team

We are all essentially social animals and, as such, need to feel a sense of belonging. We fulfil this need through our membership of a number of social groups. Our membership of a group can assume greater or less significance, depending on the situation in which we find ourselves.

Firstly, our need to make sense of the world, to impose some order on experience, leads us to categorise. We divide things into common categories such as cars, houses or trees. Then we divide them into different types of cars, houses or trees. We all do the same with people, dividing them into categories and subcategories. As with our categorisation of objects, it helps us to manage our view of the world. This may become clear if you stop for a moment and consider how you categorise the people you work with: their gender, authority, personality and so on.

Secondly, we all need to feel good about ourselves and so we look to belong to groups which nurture that feeling. When they do not, we either distance ourselves from the group or change our perception of the group so that it can boost our self-esteem. The need to feel good about being a member of a team is crucial. Think for a moment about the professional group to which you belong. How would you describe it? How important is it to you, being a member of that group? When are you most aware of being a member of that group?

A group is, however, larger than the sum of the individuals within it. Merely being a member of a group changes the way that we behave, sometimes even when we are not with that particular group all of the time. When we are in a group several things start to happen:

- we adopt *roles* within the group rather like actors in a play
- the group *develops*; it has a life of which we are a part
- we may *conform* in our own behaviour more than we would otherwise.

Each of these points will be explored in turn.

Team roles

No doubt you have amused yourself in some meetings watching the way in which individuals adopt roles within groups. There can be as many roles as there are members of the group; some people are experimenting, while others are well practised. Some will surprise you by playing different roles in one group or meeting to another, while others may stick rigidly to one particular role whatever the circumstances. We adopt roles because they come naturally to us, because we derive satisfaction from them or because others cast us in the role. Belbin (1993) identified nine key roles in work groups, which are summarised in Fig. 5.1.

Too many of one type in a team means a lack of balance; too few roles and some tasks do not get done. In a small team, therefore, one person

1. *The implementer*
   Strengths: disciplined, reliable, conservative and efficient. Turns ideas into practical actions.
   Weaknesses: somewhat inflexible; slow to respond to new possibilities.

2. *The shaper*
   Strengths: challenging, dynamic, thrives on pressure. Has the drive and courage to overcome obstacles.
   Weaknesses: can be headstrong and provoke others, hurts people's feelings.

3. *The plant*
   Strengths: creative, imaginative, unorthodox. Solves difficult problems.
   Weaknesses: can react strongly to criticism; too preoccupied to communicate effectively.

4. *The monitor/evaluator*
   Strengths: sober, strategic and discerning. Sees all options. Judges accurately.
   Weaknesses: lacks drive and ability to inspire others; overly critical.

5. *The resource investigator*
   Strengths: extravert, enthusiastic, communicative. Explores opportunities. Develops contacts.
   Weaknesses: overoptimistic; loses interest once initial enthusiasm has passed.

6. *The co-ordinator*
   Strengths: mature, confident, a good chairperson. Clarifies goals, promotes decision making, delegates well.
   Weaknesses: can perform less well with junior colleagues; delegates personal work.

7. *The team worker*
   Strengths: co-operative, mild, perceptive and diplomatic. Listens, builds, averts friction, calms waters.
   Weaknesses: indecisive in crunch situations; can be easily influenced.

8. *The completer–finisher*
   Strengths: painstaking, conscientious, anxious. Searches out errors and omissions. Delivers on time.
   Weaknesses: inclined to worry unduly; reluctant to delegate; can be a nit-picker.

9. *The specialist*
   Strengths: can make decisions based on in-depth experience, command support by their extensive knowledge of their subject.
   Weaknesses: can lack interest in other people's concerns; appears too narrow-minded.

Fig. 5.1 Belbin's team roles (adapted from Belbin, 1993).

may have to perform more than one role. The full set is most important where rapid change is involved in a service. More stable groups can cope without the full set of roles.

The leadership role is especially important. Leadership might be formally held by one individual within the group. However, the role of leadership can be and is often taken on by a number of people at different times within the life of a group (or even within a meeting). The role demands many different skills and qualities which are rarely possessed only by the formal leader and sometimes not possessed by them at all. It would be an impoverished group that did not recognise the capacity for leadership within a wide range of its group members.

Most of us have a preference when adopting a leadership role for focusing either on the task or on the maintenance of the group. This is satisfactory provided we recognise the need for a balance between task and processes within the group at any one time. It is no good focusing on people's feelings when urgent decisions have to be made, but driving through decisions regardless of people's feelings can leave a legacy of resentment.

Team development

Like individuals, groups or teams develop over time. Tuckman (1965) describes five stages through which teams can develop (Fig. 5.2).

Not all teams reach and maintain the performing stage. Most are not lucky enough to move smoothly through all phases in a neat, linear fashion. Many become stuck and many find themselves, through circumstances, moving back and forth through the same few phases. Nevertheless, to work within a team well, it will be useful for you to identify which stage of development has been reached, recognising the need to work through each stage in order to progress.

Team conformity

Being a member of a work team exposes us to social influence which can lead us to change our behaviour simply because we are a member of the group. There are at least three reasons for this conforming behaviour (Tajfel & Fraser, 1978).

- Individuals may feel that others in the group will think more highly of them if they agree with the majority view.
- Individuals may be simply agreeing for the sake of agreeing; this may be to avoid conflict, particularly if it is felt that dissent is undesirable and harmony is desirable.
- Individuals may feel overly self-conscious and uncomfortable if they stick out in a group.

---

1. *Forming*

   At this stage the group has not yet formed but is more a gathering of individuals. It is the time when parameters of group identity and activity are explored, such as its name, how often and when they will meet. It is also the time when individuals try to establish their identity within the group.

2. *Norming*

   At this stage the group tries to establish how they will work together, the level of activity and work they want to do, what is acceptable behaviour, dress, etc. These processes need not be explicit but you will be aware of them going on. For example, have you ever cracked a joke in a group and realised that this is not the sort of group where jokes are welcome?

3. *Storming*

   Inevitably, every group faces periods of conflict. These often follow a preliminary yet often false sense of consensus about the parameters of the group and its activities. As the group develops, expectations and hopes are challenged and even thwarted. This then leads to the setting of new and more realistic objectives, norms and procedures. This stage tests the level of trust that is emerging in the group.

4. *Performing*

   Only after the previous three stages of the group have been gone through, can a group expect to be effective and productive. Some groups never really achieve this level of maturity, when individuals are comfortable and committed to the group and its aims and activities. Performance even at this stage will, of course, be impeded at times by individual agendas and processes of growth (with the arrival of a new member, for example).

5. *Mourning*

   Some groups have a limited lifespan, or a significant number of members moves on and the group either folds or effectively re-forms. This can raise issues of its own for a group.

Fig. 5.2 Stages of team development.

There is a fourth reason why some one may choose to conform, based on rational rather than psychological grounds.

- They may make a judgement that, if most of the group takes a particular view, then that is more likely to be the right one, even if they disagree with it.

Teams tend to induce conformity. They curb behaviour defined as unacceptable or inappropriate, such as losing your temper. While a degree of conformity can eliminate destructive behaviour, too much conformity can stifle original or unusual ideas. What keeps the team together may not always be what gets the job done. Equally, what appears necessary to do the job may threaten to destroy the team.

Resisting team work

Finally, it is important to consider why some individuals resist team working. Katzenbach & Smith (1993) offered three reasons why people may not feel comfortable working in a team (Fig. 5.3). Such sources of resistance need to be teased out and explored. Unacknowledged, they may prevent some members making any substantial contribution to the team, which they may unwittingly seek to sabotage.

Without knowing more about the perceptions and motives of the other members of Jane's team, one cannot easily account for its apparently erratic behaviour, but some pertinent questions can be asked about the team as a group.

- How do the individuals involved feel about being part of the team?
- How are the team roles distributed within it?
- What stage has the group reached in its development?
- Why does the need to conform operate over one issue but not another?

This could be drawn out, perhaps facilitated by someone outside the group. Then, all involved would have a better appreciation of the factors governing the dynamics of the team meeting and together seek to cultivate the constructive elements and divert the destructive ones.

Teams and groups frequently function through meetings. We have explored, to some extent, the complexity of interactions which impact on the effectiveness of teams and their meetings. The effectiveness of meetings is also dependent on the extent to which the meeting is planned,

---

1. *Lack of belief in team working*
   Some people simply do not believe in team working, feeling that individuals are happier and more productive working alone. Teams appear to waste too much time talking rather than doing and seem more of a human relations exercise than anything to do with productivity. There are grounds for all of these fears. Teams can be less effective than individuals.

2. *Personal threat and anxiety*
   Sharing the control over a piece of work with others requires a level of trust and confidence in them. Working with others may seem to jeopardise both completing the task and relationships with others. Team working also exposes us to others in a way that we might find quite threatening and we will need to be confident that the team will handle weaknesses and problems sensitively.

3. *Organisational resistance*
   Sometimes the organisation itself can make it difficult for teams to work. Teams may fail if an organisation does not recognise that high performance is achieved by allowing teams the autonomy to make effective decisions and not have them subsequently overruled.

Fig. 5.3   Reasons for resisting team working.

structured and organised. Whilst details of this are beyond the remit of this chapter, some basic rules are given in the final section of the chapter.

Groups and teams are here to stay. They often present complex and sometimes uncomfortable issues; they can also be a source of a huge amount of support and creative energy. The next section addresses the issues that arise when things go wrong.

Handling difficult relationships

Understanding conflict

This chapter has already touched on potential areas for conflict at work through discussion of the team and individuals. According to Gareth Morgan (1986), conflict at work arises when interests collide:

> In talking about interests we are talking about a complex set of predisposition's embracing goals, values, desires, expectations, and other orientations and inclinations that lead a person to act in one direction rather than another. In everyday life we tend to think of interests in a spatial way, as areas of concern that we wish to preserve or enlarge, or as positions that we wish to protect or achieve. We live in the midst of our interests, often see others as encroaching on them, and readily engage in defences and attacks designed to sustain or improved our position. (Morgan, 1986, p. 149)

Each of us has personal interests that are pursued through a variety of means. These include:

- task satisfaction: our current enjoyment and satisfaction with the things that we do in our job
- career objectives: our longer term career opportunities or hopes
- extramural interests: our private values, personalities and commitments beyond the workplace.

You might like to consider your interests thinking about Fig. 5.4. How easy is it to balance the different elements? Are there any significant tensions?

We all strive to balance these three sets of interests. This is a difficult enterprise, since circumstances change around us (starting a family or children leaving home; partner starts a new job; promotion opportunities dry up; work becomes boringly routine, etc.). In the complex world of work relationships, we try to exert influence over others to achieve our own personal balance. Inevitably, conflict can arise when the interests of others do not coincide with our own; this is when political behaviour kicks in. Such behaviour is driven by the need to protect or promote our interests through the activities in which we engage at work. It is this behaviour that often leads to conflict, either overt or covert.

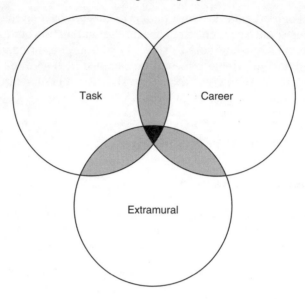

Fig. 5.4   After Morgan (1986).

Handling conflict

How, then, does one react to conflict situations? Fischer & Ury (1981) explore the dynamics of conflict. Critical to conflict resolution is the ability to stand back from the situation and try to view the issue as a problem to be solved by the parties so that each can leave feeling satisfied if not entirely happy. If you fight to win at the other party's expense, the chances are that the individual will retaliate at some later date. Fischer & Ury argue that one should aim for a win/win situation where both parties can feel good about the solution achieved. To do this, you may need to approach conflict in a way that, at first, feels strange. They suggest four strategies to resolve conflict (Fig. 5.5).

Giving and receiving criticism

The resolution of interpersonal and team conflict often involves some honest talking, including the giving and receiving of criticism, some of which is likely to be negative. This can be very difficult to handle, however confident and capable you may otherwise feel.

Back & Back (1991) outline a framework of rights and responsibilities for giving and receiving criticism (Fig. 5.6). Understanding these is vital to ensuring that such interactions are conducted in a way that is both fair and involves mutual respect.

1. *Separate the people from the problem*
   You cannot change personalities but problems can be solved. Saying that it is 'just the way they are' lets you off the hook. People's behaviour is not fixed. Someone who is very shy in meetings might be a gregarious youth group leader in the evenings. If you accept this principle, then it follows that people's behaviour at work is at least as much to do with the situation in which they find themselves ... and you are part of that situation.

2. *Focus on interests, not positions*
   Instead of focusing on the other person's position, focus on what they are interested in or concerned about. What they think may be less important than why they think that. Explore these concerns thoroughly.

3. *Invent options for mutual gain*
   In handling conflict constructively, you need to be creative. There is a real danger that you will find yourself backed into a corner if you are unable to see creative ways of reaching a solution, such as offering a compromise, discovering a new option or inviting people to air exactly why they are worried.

4. *Insist on objective criteria*
   It is important to agree on some objective criteria for judging the outcome of a resolution. There needs to be common agreement about not only which option to adopt, which can became a battle of wills, but which criteria are most relevant, which may produce more agreement. All of this requires a good deal of give and take, especially of criticism.

Fig. 5.5 Strategies for conflict resolution.

Giving criticism
- Establish that criticism is a legitimate means to improve people's performance.
- Assert the right to criticise that performance.
- Criticise in way that does not attack the person, put them down or make them look small.
- Give them the right to respond assertively to criticism.

Receiving criticism
- Clarify the nature of the criticism, if you are unclear about it.
- Do not overreact to a personal attack. Try to separate the content (which may be valid) from the way it is given. It is possible to express your unease with the way the criticism is given whilst accepting its content.
- Disagree constructively and assertively, but not aggressively, when you feel that the criticism is unjust.
- Try to find a way forward. Agree how in the future you can avoid past mistakes.
- Remain in touch through non-verbal behaviour. Try to maintain steady eye contact and keep your voice up rather than letting it sink down, so as not to show yourself to be on the defensive; this will encourage the other person to talk with you in a less attack/defence mode.

Fig. 5.6 Rights and responsibilities for giving and receiving criticism (after Back & Back, 1991).

It is easy to criticise others, but more difficult to do it constructively. It is easy to resent criticism by others, yet more difficult to appreciate its good intent.

Apparently, Jane's team successfully handled potential conflict over patient administration of drugs but did not manage this over multidisciplinary notes. The conflict over the latter may have involved different perceptions of how the proposal would affect each individual's life interests. It may also have been that the problem was not separated from the people, positions rather than interests were emphasised, options were not explored and objective criteria were not established. Finally, it would be useful to know how well the consultant, Jane and other members of the team were able to take and give criticism of their proposals.

As the example of patient administration of drugs showed, the team was sometimes capable of handling difficult issues. The team and its individual members might benefit from considering the underlying factors which led to a successful resolution of one issue but not of the other.

Conclusion

This chapter has illustrated how working with people is a complex and difficult task. It has suggested that, in order to improve working relationships, it is necessary to recognise the range of motives and perceptions driving individual and group behaviour that may not always lead to constructive outcomes.

At the level of individual interactions, we often assume that everyone involved shares the same definition of the situation and is working towards common goals, but this may not be the case. The text has also outlined ideas about the different ego states that people can unwittingly adopt when relating to others.

Working in teams presents another set of complexities. Within a team, individuals adopt roles, different in kind but each with a contribution to make. Teams should go through a series of stages in their development, although some may falter and backtrack. Teams induce conformity, which can be constructive but may also be debilitating. Teams may work less well if individuals have reservations about working in a particular, or any, team.

The final concern, handling difficult relationships, has highlighted that these may be affected by the different balance of life interests sought by team members. Constructive handling of conflict was illustrated by strategies for reaching a clear decision which all can accept. In particular, knowing how to give and receive criticism is important for interpersonal and team interactions.

These approaches have been applied to Jane's situation, suggesting how they could shed light on the behaviour which puzzled and frustrated her.

In her case, and your own working life, analysing how and why people behave in the way they do is a step on the road towards minimising conflict and maximising co-operation amongst both individuals and teams who work together.

Tips for effective meetings

This chapter began with a description of a meeting. It is possible that many of the problems encountered in this particular instance could have been helped if some basic general principles about holding meetings were adopted, whether they be staff meetings, case conferences or less formal project groups. Here is a checklist of practical things to do before, during and after meetings to ensure that they are efficient and effective.

(1) *Before the meeting*
   - Give people *sufficient notice,* preferably in writing. Organising a meeting that no one (or only some) can attend is not only disappointing and demoralising but can also waste everybody's time. It can also delay important business as the meeting must be rearranged for a later date. Ideally, arrange the next meeting at the previous one whilst people are present with their diaries.
   - Ensure that all those attending the meeting have *any documentation sufficiently in advance* that they can reasonably be expected to read it. If people attend meetings ill prepared, they can feel frustrated and discussion will suffer. Lack of preparation can also prevent members consulting others interested in the issue and so devalue the debate.
   - *Set a clear agenda.* Every group should have rules about how, when and by whom agendas are set. If every member of the group is expected to be prepared to contribute fully to a meeting, they need to have the agenda in advance and to have the opportunity to shape it.
   - *Think about how the meeting will be organised* beforehand; the process is as important as the content. The way in which things are discussed and presented will make a real difference to the motivation and commitment of those attending.
(2) *During the meeting*
   - *Ask open questions.* Rather than simply expressing your own views (important though that might be), invite others to express their view by asking questions to which they can respond.
   - *Be assertive yourself and recognise that right in others.* Do not allow others to talk you into submission, but insist that they recognise your right to disagree and express your difference of opinion without being shouted down. Equally, remember that others have the same rights as you.

- *Suggest ways of breaking the group down.* If a meeting seems to have become stuck in a pattern of interaction that is either negative or unhealthy, it may be worthwhile to suggest that the meeting be held in a different way. For example, members could split into smaller groups to discuss topics of concern, enabling those reluctant to speak in the large group to find a voice. Only the necessarily formal meeting (and there are very few of those) needs to be held in the traditional way.

(3) *After the meeting*
- Make sure that *action is monitored and a record of decisions* is distributed as soon as possible after the meeting to remind everyone of the agreements made.

References

Back, K. & Back, K. (1991) *Assertiveness at Work – A Practical Guide to Handling Awkward Situations*, 2nd Edn. McGraw-Hill, London.

Belbin, M. (1993) *Team Roles at Work*. Butterworth-Heinemann, Oxford.

Berne, E. (1964) *Games People Play*. Penguin, London.

Fischer, R. & Ury, W. (1981) *Getting to Yes – Negotiating an Agreement Without Giving in*. Arrow Books, London.

Katzenbach, J.R. & Smith, D.K. (1993) *The Wisdom of Teams – Creating the High Performance Organisation*. Harvard Business School Press, Boston, MA.

Morgan, G. (1986) *Images of Organisations*. Sage, London.

Tajfel, H. & Fraser, C. (Eds) (1978) *Introducing Social Psychology*. Penguin, London.

Tuckman, B.W. (1965) Developmental sequence in small groups. *Psychological Bulletin*.

Further reading

Hayes, N. (1977) *Successful Team Management*. International Thomson Business Press, London.

Chapter 6
Legal Aspects of Clinical Practice

Introduction

There is a wide range of legislation relevant to the practice of the therapy professions. Some of this is specific to Professions Allied to Medicine (PAMs) such as the Professions Supplementary to Medicine (PSM) Act 1960. Other legislation relates to the practice of health care, such as the Medicines Act 1968 or the Access to Health Records Act 1990. The wider legislative framework encompassed in civil law (e.g. negligence) or criminal law (e.g. indecent assault) also governs practice. Therapists are also subject to non-legislative codes such as codes of conduct, standards of care or clinical guidelines and protocols, all of which may be used in a court of law.

Increasingly, therapists are requested to write legal reports. Therapists frequently ask questions about their practice and professional liability insurance. This chapter provides an overview of the key laws that govern therapists' clinical practice and the main issues that they are most likely to face. Readers who seek more detailed knowledge around this subject should refer to other books and articles for more in-depth information.

The chapter begins by considering the PSM Act 1960, followed by Rules of Professional Conduct and issues of multiprofessional assessment and health records. Key issues of The Children Act 1989, health and safety, and consent are then explored. Finally, the chapter considers negligence and criminal actions, and provides guidance on writing legal reports.

Professions Supplementary to Medicine Act 1960

The PSM Act 1960 established the Council for the Professions Supplementary to Medicine (CPSM) as an independent, self-regulating, statutory body. The United Kingdom Central Council for Nursing, Midwifery and Health Visiting (UKCC) and the General Medical Council (GMC) are the equivalent bodies in nursing and medicine.

At its inception the CPSM covered seven professions; it now includes the following nine professions:

- art, drama and music therapy
- chiropody and podiatry

- dietetics
- medical laboratory science
- occupational therapy
- orthoptics
- orthotists and prosthetists
- physiotherapy
- radiography.

Ambulance paramedics, clinical biochemists, and speech and language therapists are expected to be incorporated in the near future, completing the 12 professions allowed under the Act. At the time of writing, the Act has recently been reviewed and major changes are expected, subject to its consideration by Parliament. Further details of the practical implications of the Act and its likely changes are given in Chapters 3 and 9.

Currently, each profession has its own Board and each Board elects a member to sit on the CPSM. Traditionally, this is the Chairperson of the individual Boards, who is a member of the registered profession. The Boards, as well as the Council, are made up of elected professionals and nominated members of Royal Colleges, educational bodies and other relevant organisations. The Chairperson of the Council is appointed by the Privy Council, to whom both the Council and the Boards are ultimately accountable.

The main function of the Council and Boards is the protection of the public and to ensure that an annual register of annual subscribing state registrants is published by each Board. To be state registered, which is a prerequisite to working in the National Health Service (NHS), a registrant must complete a course of study at a university or higher educational body recognised by the relevant Board. Both the Occupational Therapists (OT) and Physiotherapists Boards undertake this recognition with their relevant professional body, the College of Occupational Therapists (COT) or the Chartered Society of Physiotherapy (CSP). A Joint Validation Committee, consisting of members of the Education Committee of the relevant professional body and Registration Committee of the relevant Board, validates the courses leading to a recognised qualification. This gives eligibility for both membership of the professional body and state registration. Therapists who have trained overseas must apply for registration to the Registration Committee of the appropriate Board. Individual Boards vary in the processes they apply to such applicants, usually depending on the number of applicants received. For example, the Physiotherapists Board received 1000 applicants in 1997, whereas the Radiographers Board received four. Different processes may apply for EU and non-EU applicants; for example, the OT Board uses a university to examine non-EU overseas applicants.

As well as setting educational standards and producing a register, the Boards have a disciplinary function, responding to complaints against registrants. Each Board has an Investigatory and a Disciplinary Committee which processes complaints in a formal manner. Each Committee constitutes members of the Board with professional membership in the majority. This self-regulatory function, at arms' length from the professional bodies, seeks to protect the public in respect of any professional acting in an unprofessional manner that may amount to 'infamous conduct'.

Rules of professional conduct

Most therapy professional bodies such as the COT, CSP and the Royal College of Speech and Language Therapists (RCSLT) set codes of conduct against which they expect their members to practise. These codes of conduct are not enforceable by law, nor do they have formal legal standing. However, they could be used in a court of law as evidence of the standards against which therapists are expected to practise. For example, the Rules of Professional Conduct of the CSP cover a wide range of issues; not only may contravention of them amount to serious professional conduct, but a criminal or civil action could result in a disciplinary hearing, citing the outcome of that action as evidence by the complainant.

Rules of conduct or ethical codes set out the moral and ethical framework within which therapists are expected to operate. They will usually cover the following areas.

- Scope of practice is covered, as well as the need for a practitioner to establish and maintain safe and competent practice. This includes continuing professional development, lifelong learning and professional liability insurance cover.
- Therapists' relationships with patients are central to practice. Issues likely to be covered by codes include: respect for personhood, autonomy and the opportunity for information exchange; goal setting and consent to intervention; information recording and secure storage; and confidentiality, a basic and vital expectation of all patients.
- Therapists are expected to act in a proper manner in all contacts with other professionals both within and outside health care, and with carers and patients' families. The needs and expectations of multidisciplinary teams, with their focus on the patient, are also likely to be expressed within the code.
- Increasingly, therapists have a duty to report to an appropriate authority, circumstances or activities which may put the patient or others at risk. This embraces a range of issues from whistle-blowing in respect of competency to the debate regarding rationing.
- In a competitive world, therapists working outside an employed

relationship must advertise their skills, services and facilities in a way that gives the public accurate and appropriate information. Doing this in a professional but effective manner often calls for judgement which therapy professionals may find difficult. The principles of the British Codes of Advertising Practice and Sales Promotion can be of assistance here.

- Professional people are often asked to endorse, sell or promote equipment, orthotics or other related devices by manufacturers, many of whom are unaware of the codes against which therapists practice. For example, the CSP advises its members that any endorsement, selling or promoting does not exploit the patient/therapist relationship, so a therapist may sell a collar to a patient, but should only make a small handling charge. They could not recommend a particular type of splint where the manufacturer was paying them commission on the number sold; this is obvious exploitation.
- There are other circumstances where the actions of a therapist may bring the profession into disrepute, such as disciplinary action by the relevant CPSM Board or employer, conviction by a court or their own personal conduct. Any such actions could be outside codes of conduct and subject to disciplinary procedures.

As health- and social-care professionals, therapists are expected to act in a manner which brings credit not only on themselves, but also on their chosen profession.

Multiprofessional assessments and record keeping

Therapists work across a number of agencies (NHS, Education, Social Services) and in a number of health-care environments, supporting patients and clients both individually and collectively. Subsequently, in recent times, there has been increasing interest in joint methods of assessing need and recording treatment, together with joint care management plans. Increasingly, cross-agency teams are developing assessment protocols that enable the patient or client to discuss their physical and other problems with just one or two members of the team – a joint care plan is developed which constitutes the clinical record.

As information technology within the NHS progresses, the electronic health record (EHR) and the electronic patient record (EPR) will become normal practice. These will facilitate cross-agency working – further details of HER and EPR can be found in 'Information for Health'.

Health-care law

Legislation which affects therapists mainly centres on records and information, and includes the:

- Data Protection Act 1984
- Access to Medical Reports Act 1988
- Access to Health Records Act 1990
- Access to Personal Files Act 1987.

The Data Protection Act

The Data Protection Act 1984 regulates the collection, processing and storage of information in automated form, from which an individual can be identified. Anyone wishing to collect, process and store data, usually by electronic means, must register with the Data Protection Registrar. Those holding data, such as private practitioners, will need to register as individuals; in the NHS, a Trust will register as an organisation.

The Data Protection Act sets out a number of principles with which anybody holding data (electronic or paper) must comply. Data must:

- be collected and processed fairly and lawfully
- only be held for specified, lawful, registered purposes
- only be used for registered purposes or disclosed to registered recipients
- be adequate and relevant to the purpose for which it is held
- be accurate and, where necessary, kept up to date
- be held for no longer than is necessary for the stated purpose
- be surrounded by appropriate security
- be subject to a right of access by the subject of the data.

Thus, under the Act, the person about whom the information is held has right of access to the information; this includes being informed about the existence of such information and the right to a copy of the information. Children, if they are mature enough, have the same rights.

For data held as personal health records, access provisions are modified to allow health professionals to refuse access if it would be likely to cause serious harm to the physical or mental health of the data subject, or would reveal the identity of another individual, who has not consented to disclosure (i.e. who is not a health professional). For the data subject to access information held, an application is made in writing to the person or institution holding the data, together with an appropriate fee. Most Trusts have a clear policy for this process, which should be readily available. Neither the process nor the fee should prohibit reasonable access.

Access to Medical Reports Act 1988

This Act enables patients to have access to reports about them written by clinical professionals for insurance companies or employers. The Act also gives patients the right, if necessary, to suggest corrections to the report.

Access to Health Records Act 1990

The principles of the Data Protection Act, including the issue of access, apply to all records. However, despite the Data Protection Act, an anomaly existed in relation to health records: although patients could have reasonable access to records held electronically, access to paper records was denied. As most health records are in a manual form, the statutory rights laid down in the Data Protection Act had little impact for health records.

The Access to Health Records Act came into force on 1 November 1991 and only applies to records made after that date. However, access to earlier records is permitted if required to make sense of records made after 1 November.

A health record is:

- that consisting of information relating to the physical or mental health of an individual who can be identified from that information and other information in the possession of the holder of the record
- made by or on behalf of a health professional in connection with the care of that individual.

For most therapists this clearly is the clinical record made by them when assessing, treating and advising a patient (the recognised individual). A number of people can have access to this record, including:

- the patient
- a person authorised in writing to make the application on the patient's behalf
- a person having parental responsibility for a child, where the patient is a child (under 16 years of age)
- where the patient is incapable of managing his own affairs, a person appointed by the court to manage his or her affairs
- where the patient has died, the personal representative of the patient. In this situation, access can be prevented if the record includes a note, made at the patient's request, that access be denied.

Application for access to a health record or part of the health record must be made to the holder of the health record, usually a Trust. The Trust is required to seek any observations of the health professional who made the record. In the case of a private practitioner the application would be received directly. No fee can be charged unless access is requested to records made more than 40 days before the application. A charge can, however, be made for copying and postage. When an application is made, the holder of the record must allow the applicant to inspect the record or part of the record and, if requested, supply a copy or abstract.

There are exclusions where the holder can refuse access and these are similar to those for computerised records. In addition, where a person considers that any information contained in the records or part of a health record is inaccurate, they may apply to the holder of the record for the necessary correction to be made. If the holder of the record agrees, the necessary correction can be made; if the holder does not agree, a note must be made in the relevant part of the record of the matters considered by the applicant to be inaccurate. An applicant may also request an explanation of the terms used in a record. This prevents health professionals hiding behind jargon to keep information from the patient.

Access to Personal Files Act 1987

This Act applies to files held by housing authorities or Social Services. It allows access to such information in a similar manner to that for access to medical records.

The impact of all this legislation reinforces the *professional obligation of maintaining accurate, contemporaneous, comprehensive records.* Some therapists claim that excessive workloads mean that record keeping is not possible. However, records are a means of recording the care of patients; they provide clinicians with data against which they may evaluate their clinical interventions. They are part of the professional duty of care owed to the patient. *Ultimately, any clinical record can become a legal document.*

The Children Act 1989

The Children Act 1989 is the most comprehensive piece of legislation that Parliament has ever enacted about children. It draws together and simplifies existing legislation into a more practical and consistent legal code. The Act strikes a balance between family autonomy and the protection of children. In doing so, it lays specific duties upon Social Services departments, education and health-care agencies to work together more effectively in the best interests of children.

Although most of the provisions of the Act relate to legal rights and responsibilities, many principles can be extended to the therapist clinician and these must be borne in mind when working with children.

The first principle of the Act states:

> The welfare of the child is the paramount consideration in court proceedings

this principle should be applied by all therapists in their dealing with children.

The involvement of the child in decision making about their care is also a major principle of the Act. This includes the child's right to be consulted on their therapy care and treatment; children should be involved in the informed consent process as far as possible and, if competent, given total decision-making power.

Child abuse and child protection

If a therapist suspects that a child in their care, or their sibling, is being abused physically, sexually or mentally, they must take immediate action to ensure that the situation is drawn to the attention of the appropriate person. All health and local authority employers should have procedures for the management of such cases and therapists working with children must be aware of these procedures.

Where abuse is suspected, it is not always easy to decide whether action is necessary. Therapists should be aware that their main duty is to the patient or client, i.e. the child. This duty is reflected in most ethical codes and rules of professional conduct.

Health and safety

The arena of health and safety is extensive, and the following paragraphs highlight the key elements of health and safety legislation in relation to the workplace.

The Health and Safety at Work Act 1974

This Act is enforced through the criminal courts by the Health and Safety Inspectorate, which also has powers of inspection; it can issue enforcement and prohibition notices. Since the abolition of Crown immunity in respect of health and safety legislation in 1986, Health Authorities, Trusts and Social Services departments can all be prosecuted.

In 1993, new regulations came into force as a result of European Community (EC) Directives. Of these regulations, the Management and Safety at Work Regulations 1992 are the most far reaching. These apply to all work environments, and affect both employers and the self-employed. Areas of particular relevance are as follows.

Risk assessment

This is a systematic, general examination of all work and activity, to identify health or safety risks. It should not be a reactive procedure initiated after a problem or potential problem has become apparent. Associated guidance defines both risk and how risk assessment should be carried out. The process should include recording of hazards and risks, together with a statement of action and protective measures initiated. All therapists are likely to be involved in a risk-assessment process at some point.

Manual handling

Musculoskeletal injuries arising from manual handling activities are a major reason for sickness and retirement on the grounds of ill health amongst health- and social-care staff. However, only a small number of such claims are brought by therapy staff. In undertaking many aspects of clinical work, therapists are vulnerable to such injuries: they should be aware of the regulations relating to manual handling as well as the duties of the employer and of themselves in this area.

The Health and Safety Commission's booklet *Guidance on Manual Handling of Loads in the Health Services* provides specific, health service-related guidance, including information for staff working in the community. Many professional bodies have also produced profession-specific guidance which may relate to more specific issues such as for rehabilitation or the handling of inanimate loads in radiography or laboratories.

The arena of health and safety is extensive; therapists interested in further details of health and safety and its associated legislation in relation to their practice should seek more detailed documentation.

Consent

There is a considerable body of literature on consent and, most importantly, informed consent. Much of this information considers the ethical and moral duty of clinicians to ensure that their patients are kept fully informed on all aspects of their care, that is:

- that sufficient explanation is given of assessment and examination procedures and treatment and discharge activities
- that a patient's consent to these procedures is clearly documented.

The link between information exchange, consent and documentation indicates that informed consent is a process and that the clinical record should be capable of illustrating that process.

The law deals with two separate points relating to informed consent. Firstly, the duty to give information to the patient and to obtain consent could, if the patient maintains that insufficient or no relevant information was given, result in an allegation of negligence. Secondly, if consent is not received and treatment goes ahead, the patient can allege 'assault and battery' or sue for 'trespass to the person'.[1] The person who has suffered a trespass can sue for compensation in the civil courts; assault and battery is a criminal charge.

In civil cases, the victim has to prove:

- the touching or the apprehension of the touching, and
- that it was a (potentially) direct interference with the person.

The victim does not have to show that harm or damage has been done, as is required for allegations of negligence.

Most therapists' professional bodies have developed information on consent (e.g. COT, 'Statement on Consent for Occupational Therapy').

Negligence

The increase in litigation across all areas of public life has made today's therapists more concerned about being sued for negligence. Despite this, the number of allegations against therapists has not increased substantially for several years.

Negligence is defined as 'a breach of the duty of care'. It is important to note that an error of judgement may not necessarily constitute a negligent act. Accidents also happen, some of which are unavoidable despite all possible risks being considered; therefore, a patient may be harmed without this constituting a negligent act.

Four principles must be established to prove that negligence has occurred:

- that the clinician had a *duty of care* to the patient
- that there was a *breach of duty of care*
- that this *caused actual* and *reasonably foreseeable harm* to the patient.

For those employed by Trusts, allegations of negligence against an individual therapist will normally be issued against the Trust, usually by a letter of intent from the patient's solicitor or as a statement of claim. The Trust will then either appoint solicitors or use in-house expertise to seek the facts of the case. In these circumstances, the Trust will stand vicariously liable for their employee, i.e. by employing a therapist to carry out tasks on their behalf, the Trust will stand liable for that employee in the event of any allegation of negligence being made against them.

Any therapist named in such a case will be contacted by the Trust to give a statement of events. In this case, the therapist is acting as a witness of fact and the Trust's solicitor assists the therapist. It is important that the therapist involved can be identified from records and that the records are available and complete. Where appropriate, an incident form should be included. Prior to completing a report, the therapist should have access to either the letter of intent or the statement of claim, allowing them to understand clearly the allegation.

It is common for some time to have elapsed between the patient being treated and a claim being heard. Thus, records are vital to remind the therapist of the patient and allow them to report accurately and comprehensively about any incident. Trusts may need to contact therapists no longer working in their employ and should know how to contact them; in these cases, it is crucial that the therapist is adequately informed and supported.

Therapists working outside an employed situation will need to ensure that they are adequately covered for negligence associated with their practice; this is usually available through their professional organisation.

Unfortunately, negligence cases are rarely dealt with swiftly. Therapists are often left worrying about the outcome of the case for some time. Solicitors or insurers should seek to close cases as soon as possible. Many cases are not resolved or result in an out-of-court settlement. In the case of the latter, Trusts, although denying liability, choose not to go to court for a variety of reasons. In these circumstances, it is important that the therapist is involved and understands this action. Therapists often feel strongly that no negligent act has occurred and see settling as an admission of lack of competency.

A small proportion of such allegations go to court. Such cases are dealt with by the civil courts, which employ the adversarial form of procedure, but with only a judge; the burden of proof is at the level of the balance of probabilities.

Therapists accused of negligence find the situation extremely stressful. Personal support, clear information and advice should be available from both their manager and the Trust so that they fully understand the situation and the role played by solicitors and others in the process.

Legal reports

Writing legal reports

Therapists are increasingly being asked to write reports for legal purposes. (Witness of fact reports were considered in the preceding section.)

The most common type of report is that relating to a patient who is currently being or has recently been treated, e.g. physiotherapists treating a patient for whiplash injury who is seeking compensation[2] in respect of damages received from an accident; for OTs, this would be in respect

of functional ability following head injury; for prosthetists the outcome
of an artificial hub and ability to function following a road traffic accident.

The following paragraphs describe some important points to remember when writing a legal report. Therapists are usually asked to produce one of the following: a copy of notes and record of attendance; a copy of notes and/or letter of interpretation and expansion; or a report on the patient's present condition, prognosis and future care.

Request for a copy of the therapy notes and record of attendance

1. Check that the solicitor has obtained a consent note for the release of case notes. Normally, this takes the form of a signed note attached to the solicitor's letter. If this is not available, then do not release any information.
2. Look at the therapy record and refresh your memory about the case.
3. It may be that an interpretation and expansion letter is more appropriate than a copy of the patient's records if this contains shorthand references, etc. If so, suggest this to the solicitor. Be prepared to send both, along with a key to the abbreviations.
4. If notes are all that is required, simply identify relevant sections from notes and photocopy them. Enclose a covering letter with separate details of attendances, if necessary.
5. If employed within the NHS, follow the procedure of your employer. Usually, an administrator with responsibility for legal matters deals with these requests as notes are the property of the employer.
6. If you are employed, but outside the NHS, it is important to be aware of the employer's policy in respect of releasing notes, including who owns the notes.
7. If you are self-employed the decision to release notes is yours; take legal advice if necessary.
8. Ascertain whether the medical (doctor's) notes are also being sought. This is usually the case with consultant referrals, but often not so with general practitioner referrals.
9. A fee note should be enclosed, with a request for the cheque to be made payable to a specific fund (e.g. 'Therapy Fund') or employer if the associated work has been undertaken in employer's time. The fee level is usually set by employers; if you are self-employed, then the relevant professional body will usually advise.

Report on the patient's present condition, prognosis and future care

This is a request for a case report or therapy statement on a known patient (if the patient is unknown to the therapist then he or she may decline to give such a report).

1. The report should always be factual and confined to the subjects about which the therapist is knowledgeable.
2. It may be appropriate to see the patient again if some time has elapsed since the patient was last seen. This can be requested through the patient's solicitor. A charge may be made for this.
3. If the patient does not wish to be seen again, comments can be made only as to the condition of the patient when last seen.
4. The purpose of such a statement is to give *a report on present condition, prognosis and future care* and should follow the usual model for a medicolegal report, which is:
   - *history* of the injury or incident and subsequent treatment
   - *examination*, either current or at last visit
   - *prognosis*, which may include ability to work
   - *conclusion*, which may or may not include an opinion. This may include the necessity for future treatment, the requirements for care and the need for special equipment (e.g. electric wheelchair, hoist, car).
5. Agree on who is to draw up the report. Ideally, this should be the therapist who treated the patient, with assistance if appropriate. If the treating therapist has left, the report could be compiled by the clinical line manager, if appropriate. It is also useful to have the report checked before it is sent. If work is carried out in employer's time, there should be a prior agreement on fees to be charged and how the funds should be used. It may also be helpful to agree that, if desired by potential expert witnesses, independent assessments may be carried out in the department.
6. The following points are worth remembering when preparing a report.
   - Consider why a therapy report is relevant and appropriate: what does the solicitor require it for?
   - Be aware of the policy of the Trust, unit and department regarding such requests.
   - Do not give an opinion as to how the injury was caused unless this is specifically requested. It is unwise to make dogmatic statements about this unless the injury was directly witnessed; the source of any information should be attributable.
   - Distinguish carefully between facts observed yourself, information reported by others and professional opinions. Nothing should be said that would not be repeatable under oath in court. However, this does not prohibit professional judgements providing it is clear that they are such.
   - Avoid abbreviations which may be misunderstood and that are specific to a particular therapy. Adhere to 'normal' medical terminology.
   - Use a formal style.
   - Phrase the prognosis carefully with the option for reassessment at a later date if necessary. However, remember that the solicitor seeks certainty now wherever possible.

- Avoid dogmatism when giving advice about suitability for work.
- Choose words and phrases carefully, especially when offering opinions.
- Always 'sleep' on a report before sending it off.
- Do not get drawn into expressing *views* about other professions and their actions, although it may be appropriate to draw attention to matters of fact.

If writing a report or other legal work in an employer's time, permission to do so must be obtained from the relevant manager as employers are liable for work carried out in their time. In some circumstances, particularly when the therapist has done a lot of work in his or her own time, some of the fee may be paid to the therapist, but it must be declared for taxation.

Expert witness

The other type of report that therapists may be asked to write is an expert witness report. This will only apply to a small percentage of the profession, and only at very senior level. An expert witness:

- will be an acknowledged expert in a particular field and abreast of recent developments
- is there to assist the Court and not to take sides; he/she is independent and objective, although retained by one party to the litigation
- will be involved with offering opinions regarding the treatment and/or management of a case by another therapist.

An expert therapy witness may be asked to give an opinion on one or both of the following areas.

1. *Negligence*: the expert may be asked by solicitors acting on behalf of plaintiff (the patient) or the defendant (the therapist or the employer) whether another therapist's actions are negligent. It is likely that separate experts will be acting for each side. This will involve writing a report and possibly visiting council and attending court, all of which takes time and money.
2. Present conditions and prognosis and future care (*compensation report*)
    - Whether or not an employer, an insurer or an individual admits liability, a lawyer will need to quantify the cost of a claim irrespective of whether proof of negligence is required.
    - The report in these cases will involve an explanation and interpretation of the case notes, and needs to conform with the guidelines for writing a report.
    - After agreeing to give a report the therapist should or must see the

patient and any relevant medical and therapeutic notes to enable a comprehensive report to be completed.

In instances of both negligence and compensation the therapist can be required to attend court to speak on the report and can be cross-examined. The witnesses summoned to court by way of subpoena are entitled to four clear working days' notice and 'conduct money', i.e. travel by public transport from home to court. Such witnesses are obliged to attend.

If a subpoena is served on you, it is a legal document requiring you to attend court on the day eventually stated and remains valid until the case is heard. You may have to sign a document to confirm that the subpoena has been received. A court summons may also be served to require attendance at the county court; however, a subpoena takes precedence over a summons. In Scotland these are called citations.

A relevant CV should be attached to the report.

Criminal actions

All therapists must work inside the law; in fact, they are expected to practise at a higher level as health professionals. Any criminal actions taken by the police and the Criminal Prosecution Service (CPS) arising out of professional activities will normally be defended by the relevant union or professional body. This could include the appointment of solicitors for all police and other interviews and barristers for appearances in court.

Therapists who have criminal actions taken against them which occurred outside their professional activity would not normally be able to seek support from their union or professional body. However, any conviction, whether relating to professional practice or not, would be reported to the CPSM Registrar and disciplinary action could then follow. Professional bodies could also take action against a member in respect of criminal convictions.

Conclusion

There is a wide range of legislation relevant to the practice of the therapy professions, some PAMs and others relating to the practice of health care. The wider legislative framework encompassed in civil law or criminal law also governs practice. Therapists are also subject to a range of non-legislative codes.

Therapists are, on the whole, not likely to be directly involved in any civil claim or criminal case. However, they are expected to practise within the law; and comply to codes of conduct and standards of practice set by professional or regulatory bodies or their employer.

Therapists often ask questions about or seek clarification on legal aspects of their practice and professional liability insurance. This chapter addressed this with its overview of the key laws which govern therapists' clinical practice and the main issues that they are most likely to face.

Notes

1. Assault is defined as 'a threat of unlawful contact', and battery 'an unlawful touching'. Trespass to the person is 'unlawful contact or threat of contact with another person'.
2. Compensation is the award of damages for personal injury based on an assessment of pain, suffering and loss of amenity at the time, and of present condition, prognosis and future care.

Chapter 7
Aspects of Human Resource Management

Introduction

Most new or younger trained therapists will have heard of personnel departments and may have some idea of the functions that they provide. Predominantly, this will be for issues such as recruitment and selection, which they experience when they are applying for a job. However, an organisation's personnel or human resource (HR) department, as they are sometimes called, has a much wider range of responsibilities. There are many texts on these and it would be impossible to do full justice to the full range of issues and responsibilities. Thus, this chapter provides an overview of those of particular relevance to new and young Professions Allied to Medicine (PAMs).

The text begins by describing the main functions of personnel departments, going on to discuss these in more detail. Issues of recruitment and selection, manpower planning, training and development, and industrial relations (including disciplinary and grievance policies and procedures) are addressed. This is followed by details of employment contracts, payroll information and a range of other, miscellaneous issues. The terms 'HR' and 'personnel' are used interchangeably in this chapter.

The human resource function

Over recent years, many organisations have recognised the importance of the contribution made to their success and achievement by individuals. Subsequently, there is increasing interest in, and support for, the management of employees as individuals. Thus, personnel functions are increasingly being referred to as human resource management (HRM). Within the National Health Service (NHS), there has been increasing emphasis on the development of the NHS as a good employer (Department of Health, 1997); much of this development will rely on good HR practices.

HR or personnel departments are responsible for a wide range of issues, although there may be variations between organisations on the extent to which they are involved in some of these functions. These predominantly include:

- all aspects of recruitment and selection including adherence to legal requirements and organisational policies
- co-ordinating employee training and development and manpower/ workforce planning
- industrial relations, through contact with staff side organisations
- employment contracts
- a wide range of other, general issues.

The following sections describe these main roles in more detail.

Recruitment and selection

Aspects of recruitment and selection, particularly those from the perspective of the potential employee, have been dealt with in Chapter 4. However, it is important to understand the role of HR departments in this process. Their main functions are usually to co-ordinate the administration associated with the recruitment process (including organising interview panels, occupational health/medical assessments, obtaining references, etc.) and to ensure that all the relevant rules are adhered to, both in terms of legislation and in the organisation's policies and procedures (e.g. equal opportunities in sex, race and disability). The HR department often takes responsibility for issuing and monitoring employment contracts. Further aspects of employment contracts of importance to the reader are dealt with later in this chapter.

Workforce planning, training and development

As highlighted in the Introduction to this chapter, many organisations are increasingly recognising the contribution that its employees make to its achievement. Therefore, the training and development of staff and planning for future staff requirements are very important aspects of an organisation's business.

Workforce planning

In recent years, there have been significant changes to the processes within the NHS for manpower planning (within the context of the NHS, this largely means planning for the number of places at professional training schools) and the organisation of postgraduate training for PAMs. Both of these are now organised by local Education and Training Consortia, each covering around four to six Health Authorities and accountable to NHSE regional offices. Each consortium consists of managerial or professional representatives from local NHS Trusts, Health Authorities, universities/training schools and others, such as the Social Services and the private sector. The range of professions covered by each consortium may vary, but most include all PAMs and speech therapists, psychologists, pharmacists and physiological measurement technicians. Planning for some of the smaller professions is co-ordinated nationally.

Prior to the introduction of the consortia, manpower planning for each of the professions was co-ordinated at a regional level by NHSE regional offices. The consortia, via their organisation and devolved responsibility, aim to make planning more responsive to local demands. Each consortium is also accountable for postgraduate training for all professionals; previously, organised professional postgraduate training had largely been limited to medicine and nursing. Again, processes for arranging this and funds available vary within each consortium. At the time of writing, organised postgraduate training for non-medical/nursing professions remains an evolving entity.

Within organisations such as Trusts, HR departments are likely to take the lead, or at least some responsibility for, workforce planning. Again, on a practical level, some aspects of this may be managed by individual professional departments (e.g. succession planning for senior staff). However, HR departments frequently co-ordinate an organisation's liaison with its local Education and Training Consortium.

Training and development

Aspects of training and development which relate to individual career and personal development are given in Chapter 8. However, as HR departments also play a major role in training and development, some relevant issues will also be discussed here.

Whilst some aspects of training are managed by individual professional departments (e.g. through departmental In-Service Training programmes), wider aspects of this are often co-ordinated and monitored via training departments. Personnel departments may be involved in:

- organising training
- keeping records of training
- setting policies, procedures and standards for staff performance review (appraisal) and personal development plans.

Personnel departments may organise statutory training which all staff must attend on a regular basis, often annually (e.g. fire, health and safety, resuscitation). They may also co-ordinate wider, non-statutory training in such areas as computing or stress management, or recognised training such as National Vocational Qualification (NVQ) programmes.

It is not uncommon for HR departments to be an organisation's focal point for the recording of formal training and study leave. The increasing importance of continuing professional development (CPD), and the likelihood that this will become mandatory within the revised CPSM Act means that this function of HR departments may be particularly useful. At present, reports on such activity are normally available to managers.

Finally, personnel departments are commonly instrumental in setting policies, procedures and standards for staff performance review (appraisal) and personal development planning. Further details of these are given in Chapter 8.

Industrial relations

HR departments usually act as the co-ordinating point between the organisation's management and staff trade unions. The main focus for this is usually a Joint Staff Consultative Committee (JSCC; or similar title such as Joint Staffs Negotiating Committee, JNSC), where trade union representatives and senior hospital managers meet on a regular basis to discuss and negotiate around issues impacting on staff. It is normal for PAMs staff to have representation in this forum, often by their own trade union representative.

The JSCC forum deals with staff-management issues on a general level, or where they relate to particular groups of staff; they do not address issues at a personal or an individual level. However, the HR department do co-ordinate staff-management issues at an individual level. This may be in a formal way using grievance or disciplinary procedures (see below) or informally, where HR staff give independent advice or support to employees or managers.

An increasing responsibility for personnel departments over recent years has resulted from the many hospital closures, service reorganisations and mergers of Trusts, etc. Personnel departments usually co-ordinate TUPE (Transfer of Undertakings Protection of Employees) activities, the legislation which governs the transfer of staff from the employment of one organisation to another in the event of merger or transfer of services. Issues raised by these situations can be highly sensitive and require careful and thorough management. The personnel department is usually prominent in addressing TUPE issues with management and staff.

Grievance and disciplinary procedures

In any organisation, there are rules about what is deemed to be acceptable or unacceptable behaviour for both employees and employers. Some of these rules are applicable to society in its widest sense and are governed by formal legislation (e.g. an employee stealing from someone, or an employee being assaulted by a patient or even a colleague) whilst others are applicable only within the organisation (e.g. uniform standards, timekeeping and punctuality).

Every organisation will have its own grievance and disciplinary policies which set out the rules regarding what is felt to be unacceptable behaviour for employees and managers. Grievance and disciplinary procedures set out the process to be followed when an employee or a manager feels that a rule has been breached. Communicating the existence of these policies and their procedures should be included in the induction process, when commencing employment with the organisation.

Should an employee be unhappy about how they have been dealt with by a manager, they would refer to the grievance policy and would follow the grievance procedure. Where a manager is unhappy about some aspect of an employee's conduct, they would refer to the disciplinary policy and if necessary initiate a disciplinary procedure.

The exact contents of grievance and disciplinary policies and the processes involved in grievance and disciplinary procedures will vary between organisations. Their contents will have been developed and agreed with staff side representatives, usually through the JSCC and, as such, are standards generally accepted by both managers and employees. Within a grievance or disciplinary procedure, it is normal to have a number of formal stages (e.g. stage 1, verbal warning; stage 2, written warning; stage 3, final written warning), preceded by informal attempts to address the problem. For example, in a situation where an employee is being disciplined about an issue of unacceptable behaviour, it would be expected that informal attempts to address the problem constructively have been made before progressing to formal action. Only in serious cases are the more formal stages the first step in recognising and dealing with a problem.

Grievance and disciplinary procedures are relevant to both problems of an individual nature and those relating to groups of staff. Initiating either of these is a serious matter. If a therapist feels that he or she is being dealt with unfairly by their manager, they may wish to refer to the grievance policy and consider invoking the grievance procedure. However, in doing so, the therapist would be advised to discuss this with and consider the advice of their trade union or staff side representative. As part of the process, it would be expected that informal attempts had been made to address the perceived problem. Likewise, should a manager have a continued problem with the behaviour of a member of staff, then they may wish to invoke the disciplinary procedure. They would be advised to discuss this and consider the advice of their line manager and the HR department. Again, as part of the process, it would be expected that informal attempts had been made to address the perceived problem.

Employment contracts

Within the NHS, pay and conditions of service have traditionally been negotiated at national level through the Whitley Council system, a negotiating forum made up of employers and trade unions. PAMs and their related grades are represented via the negotiation body, Professional and Technical 'A' (PT 'A'), which negotiates conditions of service. Pay for PAMs is negotiated through a separate Pay Review Body (PRB).

Prior to the early 1990s, the Whitley Council/PT 'A' system was standard throughout the NHS, although it was not uncommon to see some local variation in its interpretation. However, the NHS reforms of the early 1990s brought local variations to the Whitley Council arrangements. Some of these were through enabling agreements, where nationally agreed guidance on a particular topic was issued, with the local adoption of this being optional. Others were negotiated or implemented locally. Examples include changes to salary scales, holiday, maternity or sick leave entitlement.

Today, whether employed by the NHS or by another employer, e.g. independent hospital, agency or general practitioner (GP), it is important to be clear about all the terms and conditions of service attached to an employment contract. Each will have their own rules governing their terms and conditions of employment. Table 7.1 describes some of the main questions to ask or consider.

Over recent years, in response to a number of pressures and demands on the NHS, a number of trends can be identified in changes to the conditions of service under which NHS PAMs work. It is likely these will continue or even accelerate over the next few years, as the pressures and demands of the NHS continue. Examples include:

- flexible working: part-time opportunities, evenings, weekends, annualised hours
- grading systems, e.g. the introduction of clinical specialist/assistant posts
- discretionary pay points, for those with extended roles
- more stringent monitoring and management of sickness absence
- availability of crèche and nursery facilities
- performance-related pay.

In addition, a number of external factors may influence these, not least of which is the EC Working Time Directive, which limits the number of hours that most employees can work to 48 per week.

Co-ordinating payroll information

Personnel departments are usually the interface between hospital departments and the organisation's payroll services. As such, they co-ordinate and forward information to payroll services on an employee's salary level, overtime payments, travel and subsistence payments (e.g. for attendance

Table 7.1 Employment contracts: issues to consider

Issue	Questions to consider
Salary	What is the basic salary? What are the salary scales? Any additional payments? Is there a regular increment/review? How/when is inflationary adjustment made? How/when is salary paid? Are discretionary points payable?
Holidays	What is the annual leave entitlement? Any rules around taking leave? Any additional long-service entitlements? What is the Public Holiday entitlement?
Other leave	What is the entitlement/arrangement for sick leave/compassionate leave? What is the entitlement/arrangement for maternity leave? Is adoption leave available?
On-call/out-of-hours services	Are there flexible working opportunities/ expectations associated with the job? Is there a requirement to participate in out-of-hours/on-call duties? What is the practical expectation of this? What are arrangements for recompense for this?
Pension scheme	Is there a pension scheme in place? What does it offer?
Start date/notice period	What is the start date? What period of notice is required to terminate contract by (a) employer? (b) employee?
Conditions	Is the contract subject to satisfactory (a) medical examination? (b) references?

at a course or study day), etc. They may also be the point of contact to deal with queries, errors or corrections in payment of any of the above. Details of such are usually given on the employee's payslip, which is issued when a payment is made to them, normally weekly or monthly.

Interpreting a payslip can be complicated for new employees. As well as pay information, the payslip also shows salary deductions for tax, pension contributions and National Insurance. Figure 7.1 shows a typical salary slip. Definitions of some of the sections that it contains are given below.

- *Superannuation* is the pension contribution to the NHS pension scheme. This is automatically deducted, although staff are able to contract out of the scheme and new employees are normally given the opportunity to do so. Private or other employers are likely to have their own scheme; some individuals prefer to manage their own pension requirements.
- *National Insurance* is the 'insurance' that employees pay to the government for services such as health care and benefits. It is automatically deducted from pay.
- *Tax* is the income tax paid to the government and is again deducted at source.
- *The tax code* indicates the amount that an individual is allowed to earn without being required to pay tax.
- *Gross pay* is the total salary paid before tax is deducted.
- *Taxable pay* is gross pay minus the allowance indicated by the tax code.
- *Superannuable pay* is the amount of pay against which superannuation is calculated.
- *Net pay* is the amount of money after deductions and is usually the amount paid into the employee's bank or building society account.

The arena of pay, taxation, superannuation, etc., is complex. The individual terms and conditions of employers may also vary. Thus, staff with questions about their pay or payslip should discuss them with their manager and/or personnel officer.

Pensions and other contributions

On the first day of a new job, employees are usually asked to complete a Personnel Registration form, which is likely to include a section on the pension scheme. In the NHS, employees are automatically enlisted in the NHS pension scheme unless they choose to opt out; this applies to staff who work full-time or part-time. Contributions are automatically deducted from salary.

Employees will also pay National Insurance contributions directly from their salary; these contributions are at a lower rate for those who pay into the NHS pension scheme. Under current legislation, the system will also allow payment of a state pension upon retirement [a flat-rate retirement pension rather than the State Earnings Related Pension (SERPS)].

Payroll XXX	Dept XXX	Section XYZ	Personal No. 12345	Employer XXXXXXXXX Hospital NHS Trust		Salary Scale £XXXXX	Increment Date 1st Sept	Salary / Wage £XXXXX		Standard Hours 25.00
Personal Details Miss J Bloggs				Xxxx		NI Number AB123456Z	Tax Code 123X	Gross Pay this Employment £XXXXX	Taxable Pay to Date £XXXXX	Tax to Date £XXXX
Dietetic Department				Xxxx		Cum NI £XXXX	Tax in Previous	Taxable Pay in Previous	Superannuable Pay £XXXXX	Superannuation to Date £XXXX
XXXXXXX Hospital				Job Title Senior I Dietitian						
Deductions			Amount	Pay & Allowances	Hours Worked	Hours Paid	Pay Rate		Amount	
Tax			XXX.XX	Basic Pay	25.00	25.00	XX.XX		XXXX.XX	
National Insurance			XXX.XX	Over-time	10.00	10.00	XX.XX		XXX.XX	
Superannuation (6%)			XXX.XX	Travel					XX.XX	
Staff Car Parking			XX.XX							
Staff Leisure Club			XX.XX							
				Method of Payment Bank Credit	Tax Period XX		Total Pay & Allowances		XXXX.XX	
				Date 28/11/9X	Month November		Total Deductions		XXX.XX	
TOTAL DEDUCTIONS			XXX.XX				AMOUNT PAID		XXXX.XX	

Fig. 7.1 Sample payslip.

The NHS scheme guarantees at least the same value as a SERPS and the pension is fully index linked.

Most health workers, with a few exceptions, are eligible for retirement at the age of 60 years. Exceptions include physiotherapists and mental health officers, for whom eligibility commences at 55 years.

Those who leave the NHS before pension age may be able to transfer pension benefits to another scheme. Those who join or return to the NHS late in their career may be able to transfer the value of this pension into the NHS scheme. Further details of this are given in the *Guide to the NHS Pension Scheme* (Department of Health, 1995). Those who opt out of the NHS pension scheme or are employed by a non-NHS organisation should consider alternative pension arrangements. There are many alternative schemes on offer and it would be wise to seek expert advise before choosing one of these.

It should be noted that, at the time of writing, the government is reviewing the issue of pensions; changes to current arrangements are anticipated, but remain unclear.

Other roles of the human resource department

Information recording

It is usual for personnel departments to keep confidential records of many HR-related activities. Most modern HR departments do this via a computerised system [e.g. Integrated Personnel System (IPS)]. This includes a database of employees' personal details (home address, next of kin, date of birth, start date with organisation) and a record of annual and other leave, such as maternity leave, compassionate leave or study leave. Such personal records will also include details of any current disciplinary warnings.

Staff health

Personnel departments play a significant role in the management of staff welfare. Some of this has already been raised in earlier sections of this chapter (e.g. industrial relations). However, it should be noted that personnel departments can offer support to both managers and employees in the difficult area of staff health. This can be in a preventive capacity (e.g. arranging for inoculation against diseases that employees may encounter such as hepatitis B, or ensuring provision of protective equipment) or in reaction to an issue or illness (e.g. stress associated with work or personal matters, or assistance in helping disabled employees to remain in the workplace).

Monitoring and management of sickness absence are currently of particular interest within the NHS. Within the job induction process, staff are made aware of the arrangements within their department for sickness reporting (see Chapter 4). Adherence to this is crucial to allow managers and colleagues to plan service cover for the sickness period. In general, employees must submit a sickness self-certificate (usually obtained from GP practices) for sickness of more than 3 days;[1] medical certification is required when this reaches 7 days.[1] Employee entitlement to paid sick leave is now variable both within and outside the NHS and is generally accruable, i.e. entitlement increases as the period of employment with the employer increases. Many NHS organisations allow continued service to be recognised across different employers within the NHS. Therapists should clarify sick leave entitlement before accepting a job.

In general, PAMs departments do not often exceed the standard, acceptable 4% sickness absence level. However, managers are responsible for appropriate management of sickness absence at both the departmental and individual level. Where they perceive a problem at an individual level, they may request assistance from the HR service. Personnel departments can provide assistance by arranging counselling, stress management training or referral to the Occupational Health Service or other organisations.

The wider aims of an Occupational Health Service[2] are:

- the protection of workers against health hazards at work
- adaptation of the job to suit the worker's health status
- to contribute to the establishment and maintenance of the highest degree of physical and mental well-being in the workforce (Harrington & Gull, 1992).

Hazards associated with working in a health environment may include:

- chemical hazards, e.g. contact with toxic substances, emissions into the atmosphere
- ergonomic hazards, e.g. manual handling, workstation design
- biological hazards, e.g. bacterial or viral exposure, blood-borne pathogens.

Exit interviews

In today's world, it is considered good HR practice to conduct an exit interview with employees when they leave an organisation. This provides an opportunity for the organisation or department to learn from the employees' experience of working in the establishment and to make improvements to its environment and working conditions. For many PAMs, such an interview is carried out by the relevant departmental/

professional/line manager. However, the HR department may also undertake exit interviews and this may be of value where a departing employee has had difficulties in his or her relationship with their own manager(s).

Wider human resource issues

In addition to the above roles, HR departments have responsibility for a wide range of issues throughout an organisation; these are too numerous to detail in this text. For example, an earlier section highlighted the HR role in ensuring that recruitment and selection procedures adhere to relevant legislation and organisational policies (e.g. equal opportunities such as sex and disability). However, many of these issues have wider remits which require ongoing identification and monitoring (e.g. existing staff are not being harassed or suffering as a result of their sex or a disability). HR departments have a responsibility for these issues and are likely to have been involved in the development and revision of the organisational policies and procedures.

As mentioned at the beginning of this chapter, the White Paper *The New NHS: Modern–Dependable* highlights plans to develop the NHS as a good employer. This will depend on many initiatives likely to be led, supported or co-ordinated by HR departments [e.g. flexible working, grade/skill mix changes, development of crèche facilities, CPD (see Chapter 8), career planning, 'Investors in People' and 'Healthy Workforce' initiatives].

Summary

Prior to reading this chapter, most new or younger trained therapists will have heard of personnel departments but have been unaware of the wider range of responsibilities that these departments have or of the services they may offer which may be of relevance to PAMs.

The text has described the main functions of personnel departments, issues of recruitment and selection, personnel planning, training and development and industrial relations (including disciplinary and grievance policies and procedures). Details of relevant issues associated with employment contracts, payroll information and a number of other issues have also been described. This information should better equip new or young PAMs to address personnel issues in the workplace.

Notes

1. Rules around sickness certification relate to the laws on employers' ability to reclaim sick pay from the government.
2. See the International Labour Organisation's (ILO) Recommendation No. 112 (1959) and ILO Convention 161, Recommendation No. 171 (1985).

References

Department of Health (1995) *Guide to the NHS Pension Scheme*. HMSO, London.
Department of Health (1997) *The New NHS: Modern–Dependable*. HMSO, London.
Harrington, J.M. & Gull, F.S. (1992) *Pocket Consultant on Occupational Health*. Blackwell Science, Oxford.

Further reading

Pantry, S. (1995) *Occupational Health*. Chapman & Hall, London.
Sisson, K. (Ed.) (1994) *Personnel Management – A Comprehensive Guide to Theory and Practice in Britain*. Blackwell, Oxford.
Storey, J. & Sisson, K. (1993) *Managing Human Resources and Industrial Relations*. Open University Press, Milton Keynes.

Chapter 8
Career and Personal Development

Introduction

The focus of this chapter is therapists' personal and professional development over the course of their career. As a result of today's ever-changing and increasingly complex care sector, the chapter aims to highlight the major factors that influence the personal and professional development of therapists, rather than to provide a guide to career planning.

Both personal and professional development are reviewed in the following pages. Professional development is defined as the activities which therapists undertake to ensure that they provide an ever higher quality of service and strive for the highest level of attainment and/or responsibility in their area of work. Personal development activities are defined as all other not strictly professional development activities, such as activities intended to equip therapists with skills or experience which *can* be beneficial to their practice and area of work, but directly linked to it.

The chapter also examines the changes to traditional career progression patterns over the past few years and evaluates their impact on therapists. Several broad career options are reviewed, as is therapists' progression within organisations. Finally, the chapter considers lifelong learning, as therapists become responsible for their own development and learning through continuing professional development (CPD). This includes the need to reflect on and learn from their own practice.

The points made in this chapter are generally equally applicable to qualified therapists and therapy support staff. Nevertheless, where there are important differences between the two groups of staff, these differences are highlighted. The focus of the chapter is essentially the work of therapists in the National Health Services (NHS). Again, however, many of the issues raised apply equally to other care sectors, including private practice or in Local Authority Social Services and education departments.

From career ladders to career pathways

Traditional career progression

Secure jobs with defined career pathways

The above subtitle describes two key features of therapists' jobs in the

NHS until 1990. Indeed, until then, the career of an NHS therapist was not unlike that of many other workers in large organisations of the time. Therapists were generally:

- more or less assured of holding a post for as long as they wished to practise, providing their behaviour and performance at work were not a cause for grave concern to their employers
- clear about what their career pathway, in its broad lines, would look like: the traditional grading structure (explored in a little more detail below) was seen as a career ladder; each rung on this ladder was tightly defined
- well supported by fairly extensive personal and professional networks, especially in acute hospitals.

Another general aspect of therapists' work in the past was the relatively low level of financial reward (many will argue that this is still true).

Therapy post grade definitions

The NHSE handbook (Whitley Councils for the Health Services, 1998) provides the official reference to:

- classes of therapy staff
- general definition of therapy staff grades
- specific grade definitions for each of nine groups of therapy staff.

The nine groups referred to in the section of the handbook (which deals with most of the therapy staff groups deployed in the NHS) are:

- chiropodists
- dietitians
- orthoptists
- radiographers
- occupational therapists
- physiotherapists
- art therapists
- music therapists
- drama therapists

and relevant teaching and support staff, including technical instructors. The above staff groups all come under the auspices of the Council of Professions Supplementary to Medicine (CPSM), which is the regulatory body governing state registration for these therapy professions (see Chapter 3 for further details).

Other therapy staff groups such as speech and language therapists are governed by different definitions; however, their grade structures have much in common with those referred to below. Table 8.1 shows the groups and grades for all nine groups referred to above in order of ascending seniority.

Table 8.1 Basic grading structure of the nine therapy professions

Chiropodists	Dietitians	Orthoptists	Radiographers	Occupational therapists and physiotherapists	Art and music therapists	Drama therapists
Chiropodist	Dietitian	Orthoptist	Radiographer	Occupational Therapist/Physiotherapist	Art or Music Therapist	Drama Therapist
Senior Chiropodist II	Senior Dietitian II	Senior Orthoptist II	Senior Radiographer II	Senior Occupational Therapist/Physiotherapist II	Senior II Art or Music Therapist	Senior II Drama Therapist
Senior Chiropodist I	Senior Dietitian I	Senior Orthoptist I	Senior Radiographer I	Senior Occupational Therapist/Physiotherapist I	Senior I Art or Music Therapist	Senior I Drama Therapist
Chief Chiropodist IV	Chief Dietitian IV	Head Orthoptist IV	Superintendent Radiographer IV	Head Occupational Therapist/Superintendent Physiotherapist IV	Head IV Art or Music Therapist	Head IV Drama Therapist
Chief Chiropodist III	Chief Dietitian III	Head Orthoptist III	Superintendent Radiographer III	Head Occupational Therapist/Superintendent Physiotherapist III	Head III Art or Music Therapist	Head III Drama Therapist
Chief Chiropodist II		Head Orthoptist II	Superintendent Radiographer II	Head Occupational Therapist/Superintendent Physiotherapist II		
			Superintendent Radiographer I	Head Occupational Therapist/Superintendent Physiotherapist I		
District Chiropodist: Chief II	District Dietitian: Chief II	Head Orthoptist II (District)	District Radiographer III	District Occupational Therapist/Physiotherapist II		
District Chiropodist: Chief I	District Dietitian: Chief I	Head Orthoptist I (District)	District Radiographer II	District Occupational Therapist/Physiotherapist I		
District Chiropodist: Senior Chief	District Dietitian: Senior Chief		District Radiographer I			

Source: Department of Health (1998) and Whitley Councils for the Health Services (Great Britain) (1998).

Technical Instructors are graded from Grade III (the most junior) to Grade I (the most senior). Therapy professions such as physiotherapy and chiropody also include helpers or assistants (e.g. foot care assistants, physiotherapy helpers or assistants, or occupational therapy assistants).

Table 8.1 shows that the basic grading structure is very nearly identical across all groups. The definitions for each grade vary only slightly across professional groups, and the differences relate naturally to the specificity of each job (e.g. definitions relating to occupational therapy and physiotherapy posts in places make reference to splinting or neurology; in radiography, reference is made to ultrasound work).

The grading definitions refer amongst other factors to:

- qualifications and experience
- supervision status: single-handed status, supervision duties expected or needed for the post holder to be supervised, etc.
- population served by the department in which the post holder works (for district level posts) or number of students (principal teaching posts)
- nature of the work undertaken, with precise definitions of what is meant by 'highly skilled and specialised' or 'particular expertise and ability'
- number of staff supervised and/or managed.

Prior to the creation of NHS Trusts in the late 1980s, 'District' therapy posts existed to provide a strategic element to each individual profession. These post holders were responsible for managing their entire professional group across a geographical area. As such, this could involve managing therapists in a variety of different settings, such as therapists working in several different hospitals as well as those working in the community.

The introduction of NHS Trusts, as individual employers, removed the need for such posts. More recently, individual therapy services within Trusts may be managed by senior members of their own profession and by Therapy Managers. Further details of therapy organisational structures are given in Chapters 2 and 3.

Pay scales and grades

The grade structure described above also governs the pay rates of therapists for those staff who work in NHS bodies which apply the terms and conditions of the Whitley framework. Certain NHS Trusts have adopted their own employment terms and conditions; however, such Trust-specific contracts are often closely linked to the Whitley framework, at least in relation to pay. Pay scales under the Whitley system are reviewed annually on a national basis and whilst NHS bodies have the freedom to make their own awards, they usually follow the nationally agreed awards. Pay, whilst remaining an important topic, appears to have a less high profile in today's NHS.

The changing world

Flatter structures

Organisations across the economic spectrum are generally and increasingly shedding layers of intermediary management, supervision and technical posts; this has been well documented and need not be explored at length here. The NHS is no exception to this trend and many clinical staff have felt its effects keenly. For therapy staff, on a practical level, 'flatter' NHS bodies have meant:

- the quasi-demise of the structured career ladder as a guaranteed career pathway
- for some, especially in a community setting, the sensation of isolation
- the loss or drastic reduction of old professional networks.

A fast-moving world

In addition to the above, there is an ever-increasing pace of change in the NHS which places increased burdens on all clinical staff, including therapists. Successive changes have created extra work on clinical and managerial levels, two arenas in which therapists operate daily.

One of the latest sets of NHS reforms, the *New NHS* White Paper (December 1997), subsequent consultation papers, guidance notes and other publications, and their associated developments, mean that therapists must deal with:

- clinical governance
- lifelong learning
- working with new players such as Primary Care Groups (PCGs) and later Primary Care Trusts
- new ways of assessing service and staff performance
- input to Health Action Zones and Primary Care Act Pilots
- contributing to Health Improvement Programmes.

Therapists are expected to handle and manage these new activities in the current environment and near future. Indeed, some (e.g. lifelong learning) are expected to be already in hand.

The pace of change itself over the past decade has meant some considerable upheaval for NHS staff, with subsequent impact on job satisfaction and staff morale.

Thus, it is hardly surprising that many NHS therapists do not take career planning seriously, as they perceive their future career pathways to be somewhat confused and even uncertain.

Personal and career development planning for therapists in the future

Proxy career ladders

The picture is not one of universal doom for therapists wishing to plan their careers proactively and, more generally, their personal and professional development. Much has been made in the management, human resource and therapy professional press and at conferences of the demise of the traditional career ladder. The disappearance of the traditional, structured and, to a large extent, almost predetermined career pathway is a fact of life in the late twentieth century. Although remnants of it subsist in the NHS (the Whitley framework, for instance), therapists have not escaped the consequences of successive economic downturns, combined with ever-increasing demands for health-care services.

Many replacements have been proposed for the old career ladder, including 'career climbing frames' and 'career spirals'. At the heart of such concepts are the following broad observations.

- Career progression is not necessarily always upwards; that is, it is not always in the direction of gaining more seniority and/or status and reward. Instead, sideways moves are seen to be valuable career building blocks; these can include job swaps, rotational placements and other such schemes.
- Career progression is no longer solely dependent on following structured career pathways: therapists will increasingly need to acquire power and influence to progress in their jobs through a variety of means which go beyond updating clinical skills. These can include personal development activities such as a course of study in information technology, exposure to general management activities (perhaps through the management of discrete projects), involvement in professional body special interest groups and participation in staff side activities.
- Flexibility is paramount. Job mobility is a definite trend for newcomers to the employment market. Mobility can be geographical and also sectoral: it is no longer inconceivable for not only one but several major career changes to occur in one's working life today.

Key characteristics of future personal and professional development plans

As a result, it is likely that therapists will be best equipped to plan their personal and professional development when the following conditions are met.

- They are prepared to take personal responsibility for their own professional development. This may well become a statutory requirement for the maintenance of their status as state-registered professionals in the future.
- They are prepared to make flexibility one of the key features of their plans.
- They are skilled in spotting and exploiting innovative development opportunities, which may not always represent upwards progression.

Career options

This section explores some of the key, broad activities which therapists can use in the course of their career to further their development. They include:

- specialisation in a specific clinical area
- management of therapy services or more general management activities
- careers in teaching
- research activities.

Each of these activities has its own challenges and opportunities which are not mutually exclusive. It can be easily envisaged that, in the course of their career, a therapist might be involved in all of the above, sometimes combining more than one activity in a given period.

Specialisation

Many practising therapists can justifiably claim to be specialist therapists. They may have specialised over the course of their career in working with a specific client group (e.g. people with learning disabilities), in a specific area of care (e.g. people with chronic respiratory problems) or in a specific set of procedures or interventions (e.g. rehabilitation programmes).

The process whereby therapists specialise in an area of work, and in due course become specialists, can vary from a structured career plan to an almost haphazard series of events. Many therapists will recognise their specialisation pathway as falling somewhere between these two extremes. For example, a fairly newly qualified therapist may show an interest in a particular area of practice such as community and primary care services as the outcome of different rotational posts which have consolidated their preregistration experience. They may then specialise further in this area and seek posts that give them further exposure and experience. As their specialisation increases, they offer clinical supervision, advice and support to other therapists wishing to specialise in community care and may carry out some teaching via the supervision of student therapists or in other community settings. This, in turn, helps to consolidate their practice through reflection and application of research and other findings.

This typical pathway could deviate at several points, e.g. the therapist may have a career break and on return to work may not be able or willing to return to their initial speciality. External events could intervene, e.g. a therapist could be employed in an organisation which merges with another, with the result that the combined therapy services need to be reconfigured without the therapist's continued specialisation being possible. As this latter example shows, therapists are not always able solely to determine whether and how they specialise. This is rightly the case: while therapists are in a relatively strong position in the care labour market because of the relative national shortage of therapy staff, services provided should meet patients' and clients' needs first and foremost, not primarily therapists' career goals. A therapist determined on a specific course of specialisation may need to deploy considerable flexibility to meet their objective, such as being prepared to relocate several times to attain posts most suited to their purpose.

Perhaps paradoxically, specialisation can also be argued to go hand in hand with 'genericisation'. The therapy press, papers and conferences have devoted much time and space to the debate on the desirability or undesirability of 'generic therapists', multidisciplinary education and training programmes at preregistration and postregistration levels to produce more multiskilled therapists, the fine differences between the terms 'multidisciplinary' and 'interdisciplinary', and so on.

This chapter does not aim to enter this debate but a link can be made between genericisation of therapy professionals in conjunction with specialisation of their skills in a particular area. For example, therapy rehabilitation professionals would be highly specialised in rehabilitation techniques and procedures, but generic in the sense that they would become rehabilitation therapists rather than rehabilitation speech and language therapists, physiotherapists and occupational therapists. A diabetes practitioner (who could conceivably be a nurse or a podiatrist, for example) is another illustration of this type of development, which is occurring more commonly but is not yet widespread.

Therapists keen on specialisation in their career should take note that:

- specialisation is not always possible in their area of choice, unless they are prepared to deploy flexibility
- specialisation can mean substituting their identity as therapist from a particular discipline with one as a generic therapist specialising in a particular area.

Management

For clinical staff, management as a career may seem a daunting prospect.

Whilst many therapists embrace it enthusiastically, some are suspicious of its suitability to their work ethos and culture, and lack confidence about their skills in management.

It is widely recognised, however, that in today's NHS and especially in the context of ever flatter organisations with fewer dedicated managerial layers, some degree of management is likely to form part of all therapists' careers.

So, how well are therapists equipped to cope with the challenge of management? The answer to this question depends largely on what is understood by the term 'management' (this is explored further in Chapter 1). A simple definition might be the deployment of resources, human, financial and other, to meet an objective, in this instance, provide patient/client care. Qualified therapists can all be regarded as managers as they are largely independent practitioners, managing their own caseload and time. Other management activities in which therapists may be involved include:

- staff management: managing other therapists or other staff
- budget management: managing their department's budget or part of it
- taking part in Trust, Health Authority or PCG management activities, such as attendance at planning meetings and project management.

Today, most preregistration courses for therapists include an element of management and the skills that qualified therapists may be required to deploy; some contain some basic management modules. Many therapists complain, however that they learn about management 'on the job' rather than in a structured way, and deficiencies are often identified in:

- business planning
- financial analysis
- negotiation skills.

A number of development mechanisms exists for therapists wishing to improve their management competencies, either because they wish proactively to orientate their career towards management or because they and/or their employer believe that their work would improve as a result of such development. Development mechanisms may range from in-house short courses, through peer support and employer-led management development programmes, to formal courses provided by the higher education sector or other education and training providers, including Masters in Business Administration, Certificates in Management Studies or National Vocational Qualifications.

Therapists have become managers at senior levels of NHS organisations, including Board level. When they reach this level of management seniority, they frequently give up their therapy practice, although there is no rule about this; many simply find that the demands on their time do not allow them to combine senior management posts and an active caseload. However, many therapists successfully combine managerial activities with therapy practice on a day-to-day basis. In all cases, therapy managers take a proactive stance in developing their managerial competence and capability.

Teaching careers

Pursuing a career as a therapy tutor or teacher probably has many points in common with developing a specialism in a particular area of therapy practice. That is, the move to embracing an academic career can result from a combination of planned career progression and more haphazard events.

Teaching occurs at many levels for therapists:

- teaching can be and often is an integral part of therapy practice as therapists teach patients/clients and their carers
- qualified therapists offer teaching to support staff and to therapy students in clinical placements or fieldwork experience
- therapists teach others through mentorship schemes, clinical supervision and peer reviews
- therapists can acquire the specialist skills required to teach preregistration and postqualification students.

Teaching now generally takes place in higher education institutions, especially since the mergers in recent years of old NHS Schools of Radiography, Occupational Therapy and Physiotherapy with universities. The formal qualifications required to hold academic posts are generally state registration in the appropriate profession and a higher education degree, sometimes in education; relevant clinical experience is also expected of aspiring therapy tutors and lecturers. Many therapy lecturers continue their formal education with Masters and Doctorate degrees.

Research activities

Research activities cannot be properly described as a career pathway; they are often combined with other therapy activities, notably teaching or developing a specialist skill. Indeed, it can be argued that every therapist, from the moment they qualify, has a duty to embrace research activities throughout their career.

Therapy research can take different forms and require more or less skill, experience and time. For example, therapists can be undertaking research when they:

- prepare and write their dissertation in the final year of their preregistration course of study

- take part in an audit or similar activity
- write an article for publication in a therapy professional journal
- bid for and manage or contribute to a clinical research programme in their organisation
- undertake a PhD or MPhil course of study.

Therapists have a duty to undertake research activities to fulfil the statutory duty to keep clinical skills up to date and therefore maintain state registration. At the time of writing, it is likely that this duty may become more formalised, as a result of the review of the Professions Supplementary to Medicine (PSM) Act. The concept of evidence-based practice is well established for therapists (and other care staff); if therapists' work is to be evidence based, they must be able to apply and understand the latest research available, as this represents the most current evidence. When therapists become producers of research rather than simply users of it, they contribute to the body of evidence to be used by others in the future.

Career milestones and development support

As highlighted previously, the career pathways in today's NHS are far more fluid and less structured than in the late 1980s; however, it is still possible to distinguish several milestones in a therapist's development at work. Examples include:

- their first therapy post and the induction and training that accompanies it
- taking on new responsibilities
- returning to practice for those therapists who have chosen a career break.

Each broad stage requires different types and levels of development activity by therapists and support from employing organisations. This development support is the focus of this section.

The newly qualified therapist

The first few months and at least the first year of a qualified therapist's career are essentially devoted to consolidating experience and knowledge. Newly qualified therapists (often referred to as junior or basic grade staff) rarely work unsupervised and usually benefit from a highly structured in-service training and development programme aimed at exposing them to different types of work. They also benefit from an induction programme, which aims to ensure that new staff members find their place in the organisation as quickly and as smoothly as possible (see Chapter 4 for further details).

The in-service training programme for newly qualified therapists is typically conducted through a rotation programme. In this scenario, each newly qualified therapist works for several months in different hospital departments (work in a community setting, which largely requires independent practice, is usually reserved for slightly more senior staff). As they gain experience, they may start to work with support staff and student therapists, at first under the supervision of a more senior colleague and gradually offering that supervision themselves to staff and students. At the outcome of their consolidated training period, they are deemed to be independent practitioners ready to gain further skills and possibly specialise in a specific area of practice.

Individual performance review

Therapists working in NHS organisations (and elsewhere) are generally offered individual performance reviews (IPRs; sometimes referred to as appraisal) throughout their career. These usually occur at least annually and involve the therapist and their line manager. The purpose of the IPR is to:

- chart the progress of the therapists against their work and practice objectives in the period considered
- review and discuss any areas of concern and agree a course of action to improve these
- determine any training and development needs
- agree the next set of work and practice objectives.

A good IPR should not focus on specific operational issues (although reference can be made, perhaps to illustrate a point); these should be managed as they arise, rather than stored for an unhelpful confrontation during the IPR. Instead, the IPR should be a positive performance management tool of benefit both to the therapist, in terms of their personal and professional development, and to the employing organisation. This is done by seeking to match the skills, experience and development needs of the former with the service needs of the latter, and also by encouraging therapists continually to improve their practice and job performance.

Mentorship

Another useful development tool for therapists is the concept of mentorship. Mentorship can be seen as akin to supervision, as one therapist draws on the experience of a more senior colleague. A key difference between mentorship and supervision is that the latter generally refers to clinical supervision, whereas the former can relate to all aspects of a therapist's job and not just their clinical practice.

Mentors can offer real support and pave the way for structured development for therapists by:

- offering them advice and help drawn from their specialist area of expertise and/or from their longer experience of working in NHS or other organisations
- establishing a relationship of support, perhaps through regular review meetings (which would have an objective different to IPRs and thus be separate)
- encouraging the therapist to reflect on their practice and help them to structure their thinking
- taking an interest in and promoting the therapist's training and development activities, perhaps by discussing and suggesting possible courses of study or other training and development activities.

Return to practice

A career break option is chosen by many therapists for a variety of reasons, including starting a family, looking after dependants, choosing to explore an alternative career, and working or travelling abroad. Many employers are keen to attract potential returners to practice as they have valuable skills and experience which can be (re)deployed in the NHS. Return to practice makes economic sense too, considering the high cost of training therapists borne by the NHS and the relative waste of this investment if therapists who have taken a career break never return to practice.

Returners to practice require specific support. In particular, they may experience anxiety about updating their clinical skills and coping with changes which have occurred in the organisation since they left. Tailored training and development programmes, often in the shape of refresher courses, can go a long way towards equipping returners with the skills and confidence to practise again in their chosen field. Many professional bodies play an active role in helping service managers and returners, sometimes in partnership with a higher education institution.

Lifelong learning

Continuing professional development

Earlier, this chapter described how therapists increasingly need proactively to plan their own personal and professional development. The chapter has also reviewed some of the support mechanisms that exist to help with this. This section more closely examines the concept of CPD, probably one of the largest challenges facing the therapy professions today, but one for which they are well prepared.

CPD and other terms such as continuing education are current 'buzz words'; however, the concepts that they describe have been well understood and at least partially implemented for a number of years. CPD is a part of the wider lifelong learning concept and is at the heart of some government policies currently being introduced.

What is continuing professional development?

A working definition of CPD is provided in the government's consultation paper (Department of Health, 1998) on quality, clinical governance and related activities:

> Continuing professional development (CPD) is a process of lifelong learning for all individuals and teams which meets the needs of patients and delivers the health outcomes and healthcare priorities of the NHS and which enables professionals to expand and fulfil their potential.

As this definition indicates, CPD is a lifelong learning concept and, as the whole of the consultation paper shows, is a key component of the government's intended overall framework for ensuring that high-quality services are delivered in the NHS, especially through clinical governance. The concept of clinical governance is also new; it is defined in the above document as:

> a framework through which NHS organisations are accountable for continuously improving the quality of their services and safeguarding high standards of care by creating an environment in which excellence in clinical care can flourish.

A comparison of the two definitions clearly shows the critical contribution which CPD is expected to make to clinical governance.

Continuing professional development and professional bodies

In recent years, the therapy professional bodies have been active in formulating CPD strategies and position statements. A significant driver for this has been the review of the PSM Act, currently underway, which is expected to require therapists to demonstrate CPD commitment and activities (probably on an annual basis) as a condition of maintained state-registered status. This is similar to the process already in place for speech and language therapists, a profession not regulated by the CPSM. Since 1991, speech and language therapists have been required to present a countersigned, personal, auditable log describing CPD activities, to ensure continued registration with their professional body. The current requirement of the Royal College of Speech and Language Therapists is a minimum of 10 sessions (for full-time staff; pro rata for part-time staff) of CPD activities, which are closely defined by the College.

It is likely that the PSM Act review will result in similar mechanisms existing for the professions regulated by CPSM. Although other therapy professions do not have any mandatory requirement for their members to undertake CPD activities at present, this does not mean that CPD does not exist. All of the professional bodies have policies, guidance, position statements or similar for their members which sometimes incorporate CPD in professional standards or codes of practice.

Continuing professional development and therapists

Various definitions and guidance documents make it clear that responsibility for CPD lies with different NHS players and importantly with therapists themselves. CPD formalises the process and need not represent a great cultural or practical change for therapists. However, it is clear that the government, academia and the professional bodies rightly see that CPD means more than simply keeping clinical skills up to date. A part of lifelong learning, it also means developing a framework for continuous improvement, in all spheres of therapy practice.

Reflective practice

What is reflective practice?

Reflective practice is increasingly being seen as an important cornerstone of therapists' and other care professionals' education, training and development. It is at the heart of many preregistration therapy course curricula and is often combined with problem-solving techniques to encourage students to apply their thinking to realistic situations. It is also key to care professionals' CPD, as therapists are constantly encouraged to assimilate and consolidate their cumulative work experiences by reflecting on them in a structured way and to apply the results to future work experiences and events.

Reflective practice and action learning

A similar concept to reflective practice is that of action learning, which is used in non-care professions. Action learning encourages managers and others to problem solve and learn about problem solving at the same time. Rather than use case studies or other relatively artificial learning tools, a real problem is worked through, both to achieve a positive outcome and to reflect on how to handle the problem. Action learning typically happens at group level in an action learning set, which usually has input from an external facilitator. Reflective practice, by contrast, more usually describes the learning process of an individual. Both processes rely on self-direction (even if a facilitator is present) to prompt the learner to think through and apply the results of this thinking to their practice or job.

Summary

The development of flatter organisational structures has resulted in changes to the traditional, structured career ladder for therapists and created a sense of isolation for some staff; there has also been a loss of traditional professional networks. Career spirals, with lateral organisational moves, may replace the traditional career path with more creative options. Therapists may wish to acquire more power and influence to progress in their jobs, in addition to skills updating. Flexibility, in both skills and geographical movement, is a key requisite in the current labour market.

Therapists need to take personal responsibility for their own professional development. The four main activities which therapists choose during their career are clinical specialisation, management, teaching and research. Therapists can activate management development at a range of levels from managing their own caseload to managing extensive staffing and other resources. Different mechanisms exist to upgrade management competencies and capabilities. Research should be a necessary part of a therapist's work and can take a variety of forms. Specialist research therapists enrich the body of evidence on which therapists base their future practice. Teaching can occur in a variety of situations ranging from supervisory activities to preregistration and postregistration lecturing.

Support for career development may involve a variety of initiatives including IPR, mentorship and return to practice schemes. CPD and reflective practice can be seen as vital foundations to a therapist's career and may be essential as a consequence of the PSM Act review.

References

Department of Health (1998) *A First Class Service – Quality in the NHS*. HMSO, London.
Whitley Councils for the Health Services (Great Britain) (1998) *Professions Allied to Medicine and related grades of staff (PT 'A' Council) Pay and Conditions of Service Handbook*.

Chapter 9
Professional Organisations

Introduction

This chapter presents and discusses a group of organisations which are collectively, and somewhat loosely, referred to as 'the professional organisations'. These organisations are key players in the delivery of therapy services to patients and clients within and outside the National Health Service (NHS). They are major contributors to therapists' training, development and professional support, and contribute significantly to therapy policy development at a local, regional and national level; some also fulfil a trade union function. Clearly, professional organisations are vital and powerful institutions, given their primary purpose of guaranteeing safe care delivery (with their accreditation powers) and their aims to promote the highest possible quality of care and support and development for their professional members.

Despite this, their role is sometimes unclear to stakeholders in therapy services. Between them, they can offer a fairly bewildering range of services to professionals and very little can be found which is really common to all therapy professions; this makes it a little difficult to generalise about and analyse their role. This chapter aims to shed light on this complexity and, in particular, identify areas which are common, comparable or different across organisations. The chapter discusses the key roles and functions of professional organisations both from the viewpoint of the therapy practitioner and from the broader perspective of the UK care sector. It also analyses a number of topics related to the role of therapists and their professional organisations which are the result of recent change or subject to impending change.

The chapter has the following structure:

- What is a professional organisation?
- Spectrum of services offered
- State registration and the review of the Professions Supplementary to Medicine Act
- Professional organisations as trade unions
- Professional organisations as accrediting bodies
- Definers of professional standards of practice and codes of conduct
- The future for therapists' professional organisations.

What is a professional organisation?

A multiplicity of terms to describe 'professional organisations'

Devising a comprehensive list of all professional organisations associated with therapy groups and other non-nursing/non-medical care professions would be a time-consuming task; a detailed description of these is not the focus of this chapter. Instead, it will discuss several key features of therapists' professional organisations, drawing on specific examples to illustrate particular points. The more specific aim of this section is to attempt a definition of a professional organisation and an explanation of the types of service that these organisations can offer.

The following expressions and terms applied to different organisations will be found throughout this chapter:

- associations
- trade unions
- accrediting organisations
- colleges
- councils
- societies.

These terms are a clear indication that a variety of roles is fulfilled by organisations that represent therapists in one form or another. Yet the word 'represent' does not adequately describe the key functions of professional organisations taken in their broadest remit, as it only describes part of their activities and services. A glance through some of the literature provided by different therapy organisations provides the following examples of objectives pursued, definitions or terms of reference:

to promote and develop for the public benefit the science and practice of radiography and therapeutic technology and allied subjects (Society of Radiographers).

It is responsible for setting, promoting, and maintaining high standards in the education, clinical practice and ethical conduct of speech and language therapists (The Royal College of Speech and Language Therapists).

... the Association has developed into a professional association which aims to:
- inform
- protect
- represent
- and support
its members (British Dietetic Association).

The Society performs three important functions for our members concerning the roles of professional organisation, educational body and independent trade union (Chartered Society of Physiotherapy).

'Representing' members, then, is a key function of professional organisations, although not the only one, as these examples show. Implicit or explicit in the above statements is the notion that the care provided by therapists can be a matter of public safety. Some organisations therefore have as a key concern the protection of the public, which can be described as a continuum, encompassing the promotion of the highest possible standard of therapeutic practice at one end and the protection of the public against potentially dangerous, or even fatal, effects of poor practice, at the other.

The word 'standard' is another frequent feature of mission statements or definitions of purpose; it is often found in the expression 'professional standards of practice' and represents another key element of professional organisations' work. Defining these standards and drawing a code of conduct for the therapist members is clearly closely linked to protecting the public and promoting the development of ever higher standards of therapeutic care.

Proposed definition of a professional organisation

The paragraphs above have shown that different words describe organisations which deal with professional matters for therapists. In the subsequent sections in this chapter, the expression 'professional organisation' will be taken to be a generic word for such organisations. The Chartered Society of Physiotherapy, the British Association of Occupational Therapists and the College of Radiographers are all examples of professional organisations.

As mentioned previously, whilst generalisations are difficult in relation to professional organisations, the following definition is proposed:

> Professional organisations for therapy groups represent their members, who are therapy practitioners; they contribute to the protection of the public and also promote practice development for the benefit of the care sector as a whole.

Membership and organisation: a brief outline

The membership of therapy professional organisations consists, in the main, of practising therapists (although a number of members may no longer be actively practising). A condition of membership is often registration with the appropriate organisation, usually the Council for Professions Supplementary to Medicine (CPSM), which is reviewed in more detail later in this chapter.

Professional organisations are largely funded through the fees which they levy from their members. Fees depend on such factors as the length of membership period, the seniority level of the therapy practitioner, status as a practising therapist, the level of insurance cover and subscription to a professional journal.

The management, leadership, structure and organisation of these associations take different forms.

- Specific activities are managed by individual senior officers employed by the organisation.
- Some organisations have regional offices.
- The senior management team often forms a Council.
- Boards and committees fulfil specific functions (e.g. an ethics committee or an academic board).

The above list is not exhaustive and the range of different management arrangements and organisational structures and processes is another illustration of professional organisations' diversity.

The legal status of professional organisations is another variable factor: some are registered charities (e.g. the British Dietetic Association), others are companies (the British Association of Occupational Therapists Ltd and the College of Occupational Therapists Ltd) and the Chartered Society of Physiotherapy is incorporated by Royal Charter.

Spectrum of services offered

Range of services offered

Table 9.1 attempts to provide an indicative list of the types of service offered by different professional organisations. For illustrative purposes, it indicates which organisation provides what services to its members (be they in the public, private or independent sector), to the NHS and to the public. Additional services to those mentioned in Table 9.1 include:

- publication of information leaflets and packs
- organisation of and contribution to regional, national and international conferences
- library services and information telephone hotlines
- income generation activities such as hire of conference facilities, and sale of publications and merchandise.

Diversity of arrangements

Table 9.1 shows that the services offered to members vary from organisation to organisation. Some professions have two organisations concerned with professional matters, each offering a different type of service, such is the case for occupational therapy and radiography. The British Association of Occupational Therapists (BAOT) and the Society of Radiographers (SOR) can be described as associations of therapy professionals, whose main purpose it is to represent the interests of their members. They may be active in pay negotiations with the Pay Review Body, for example, and offer their members professional indemnity insurance. For these two professions, accreditation of courses leading to a qualification attracting state-registered status, the definition of professional standards of practice and other related activities are the more specific remit of the College of Occupational Therapists and the College of Radiographers.

The Chartered Society of Physiotherapy, the British Dietetic Association and the Society of Chiropodists and Podiatrists, however, offer all the services which the BAOT and COT or the COR and SOR together offer. The Royal College of Speech and Language Therapists (RCSLT) is different again; this professional organisation has the power of registration for this group of professionals, whereas all other professions mentioned in Table 9.1 (and also orthoptics, medical laboratory science, orthotists and prosthetists) come under the registration authority of the CPSM. The role of the CPSM in relation to state registration is explained below and in Chapter 2.

State registration and review of the Professions Supplementary to Medicine Act

The Council for Professions Supplementary to Medicine and its role

The CPSM is the organisation which confers state-registered status to therapists and other professions (and which is a condition of employment in the NHS). The CPSM is a federation of independent, self-regulating organisations comprising one Board for each of the professional groups whose members are likely to seek registration, the Council itself and the Privy Council. The Privy Council has default powers of intervention, similar to other professional organisations, to be carried out in the event that the CPSM was not performing its duties adequately. At the time of writing, nine professions fall within the terms of the Professions Supplementary to Medicine (PSM) Act:

- arts (arts, music and drama) therapy
- chiropody
- dietetics
- medical laboratory science

Table 9.1 Range of services offered

Services offered by some professional bodies for therapists	State registration	Accreditation and joint validation of education and training courses	Indemnity insurance	Pay negotiations	Other industrial relations services/ representation of members	Definition of professional standards of practice and code of conduct	Professional/ career advice and/or support	Promotion of research and development
Chartered Society of Physiotherapy	No (state registration via CPSM)	Yes	Yes	Yes	Yes (CSP is affiliated to the TUC)	Yes	Yes	Yes
British Association of Occupational Therapists (BAOT)	No (state registration via CPSM)	No (see COT)	Yes	Yes	Yes (links with UNISON)	No (see COT)	Yes	Yes
College of Occupational Therapists (COT)	No (state registration via CPSM)	Yes	No (see BAOT)	No (see BAOT)	No (see BAOT)	Yes	Yes	No (see BAOT)
Royal College of Speech and Language Therapists (RCSLT)	Yes (speech and language therapists have to register annually with RCSLT)	Yes	Yes	Yes	Yes	Yes (published in *Communicating Quality*)	Yes	Yes

(Continued overleaf)

Table 9.1 Range of services offered (continued)

Services offered by some professional bodies for therapists	State registration	Accreditation and joint validation of education and training courses	Indemnity insurance	Pay negotiations	Other industrial relations services/ representation of members	Definition of professional standards of practice and code of conduct	Professional/ career advice and/or support	Promotion of research and development
College of Radiographers (COR)	No (state registration via CPSM)	Yes	No (see SOR)	No (see SOR)	No (see SOR)	Yes	Yes	Yes
Society of Radiographers (SOR)	No (state registration via CPSM)	No (see COR)	Yes	Yes	Yes (SOR is affiliated to the TUC)	No (see COR)	Yes	No (see COR)
British Dietetic Association	No (state registration via CPSM)	Yes	Yes	Yes	Yes	Yes	Yes	Yes
Society of Chiropodists and Podiatrists	No (state registration via CPSM)	Yes	Yes	Yes	Yes	Yes (the Society is affiliated to the TUC)	Yes	Yes

Notes to table are given below.

Table 9.1 Range of services offered (continued)

State registration: see text.

Accreditation and joint validation of education and training courses: see text.

Indemnity insurance: all therapy professionals can avail themselves of this from the relevant organisation and the insurance premium forms part of the membership fee. This insurance protects therapists against alleged claims of negligence, up to a certain sum, e.g. one million pounds; this is known as professional indemnity insurance. Retired therapists can also take out insurance to protect them against claims potentially arising out of actions when they were practising, usually for a lesser premium. Some professional organisations also offer an additional service insurance against personal accidents.

Pay negotiations: many professional organisations have an active lobbying role in this area. Most therapy professions and non-nursing, non-medical clinical professions in the NHS are paid according to the PT 'A' salary scales enshrined in the Whitley Council framework. The main pay negotiation channels are via the national Pay Review Body to which organisations such as professional organisations make representations.

Other industrial relations services/representation of members: see text.

Definition of professional standards of practice and code of conduct: see text.

Professional/career advice and/or support: many therapists turn to their professional organisation when they require specialist professional support. They do this in a variety of ways: by contacting the relevant committee, board or special interest group to which their query relates; by contacting a general information department as their first port of call; by attending conferences and seminars organised by their professional organisation, etc. Some organisations are also able to offer financial assistance via their benevolent fund to members experiencing real hardship.

Promotion of research and development: a profession that is active in research and development activities, and is successful in applying findings in new care pathways and modalities, is one which seeks to extend the scope of its practice and define ever higher standards of care. Promoting research and development is therefore seen to be a key activity of many professional organisations. This can take the form of research strategy formulation, interprofessional co-operation, collaboration with the education sector, support to therapy members with advice on research methodology and access to libraries and other resources, or the award of research bursaries.

- occupational therapy
- orthoptics and orthotics
- physiotherapy
- prosthetics
- radiography.

As well as conferring state registration to practitioners and maintaining a register of state-registered professionals, the Boards and, in particular, their investigating and disciplinary committees, conduct disciplinary proceedings, although these are currently in the main confined to allegations of 'infamous' conduct. The Boards also have the important function of approving courses and examinations to ensure that new graduates are fit for practice (see below for more details on course accreditation and validation). Further details of the CPSM are given in Chapter 2.

Review of the Professions Supplementary to Medicine Act

The PSM Act 1960 is currently being reviewed and new legislation debated. A review has been conducted by an independent organisation commissioned by the NHS Executive on behalf of the four UK Health Departments. Following a large-scale consultation exercise, a report has been published.

Some of the key changes proposed concern setting up a single regulatory organisation, rather than individual organisations for each profession and updating disciplinary procedures. Other important changes concern the proposed protection of title for therapists and other professions; this would ensure, for example, that only a duly state-registered occupational therapist could used the title 'occupational therapist' when exercising their functions. Arrangements would need to be made for those practitioners who do not meet the state-registered criteria (there is a number of these, for instance in the chiropody profession).

State registration and continuing professional development

Another important change is the stronger emphasis on continuing professional development (CPD) for professionals. New legislation has yet to be drawn up, so it is not certain at the moment that CPD will be mandatory in order to maintain state registration, but it is safe to say that CPD is to gain increasing importance for therapists. Assuming that CPD becomes mandatory, questions immediately arise about what form it will take and how it will be monitored. It is likely that individual professional organisations will have a key role to play in these areas, thus reinforcing the principle of professional self-regulation which is at the heart of the PSM Act and is guiding its review. One possible outcome of the PSM Act review may be the requirement for individual therapists to provide evidence that they have kept up to date, via an individual development portfolio. Reregistration may be dependent on presentation of such evidence, and clearly the CPSM could have a role to play in this area.

Professional organisations as trade unions

Trade union activities of professional organisations

As mentioned above, the radiography and occupational therapy professions have each set up two organisations to represent their members. BAOT has established a link with UNISON: when therapists become members of BAOT, they automatically join UNISON. SOR is affiliated to the Trades Union Congress. Neither BAOT nor SOR can accurately be described as a trade union, yet they both offer certain services that might be expected from trade unions. They could perhaps be termed 'associations' to differentiate them from their College counterparts (COR and COT).

Types of service offered

The types of service which professional organisations offer in a 'trade union' role, whether the organisation primarily functions as an 'association' or it is an organisation which encompasses this role alongside other services, can broadly be defined as support and representation. These services often include:

- support and representation of members in the case of a claim before an industrial tribunal, e.g. for sex or race discrimination, or unfair dismissal
- support and representation of members in disciplinary procedures
- trade union support in places of employment, such as hospitals, through a network of stewards and elected officers
- advice on health and safety issues and other employment issues.

Professional organisations as accrediting bodies

Accreditation of preregistration education and training programmes

Most care professionals, and certainly therapists and members of staff from Professions Allied to Medicine (PAMs), undergo a period of education and training prior to gaining state-registered status, where such a status exists (this is the case for the major therapy professional groups: physiotherapists, occupational therapists, radiographers, dieticians, etc.). The successful completion of the course of undergraduate study, which comprises both academic and clinical components, leads to state registration and enables entrants to the professions to start their career as qualified workers. Qualified professional staff are distinct from their support worker colleagues (helpers, therapy assistants, technicians, etc.) who, although they may have undergone formal education and training courses, are not state registered.

Clearly, the responsibilities of the providers of education and training courses which are conditional to students becoming state-registered professionals (these courses are often referred to as preregistration courses) are significant. However, providers of education and training do not shoulder the responsibility of the type, structure and quality of the preregistration courses, as these are vetted by the professional organisations, by the CPSM and others involved in the course accreditation processes.

Professional organisations keep a register of establishments where accredited courses are run; they have a rolling programme of inspection and reaccreditation and generally fulfil a quality-assurance role. To help undertake accreditation, organisations work with education and training providers and NHS partners, who are key players in the clinical components of preregistration courses, providing staff and resources for clinical placements.

Accreditation is usually the remit of a particular group within a professional organisation, with specific responsibility for education and training matters, e.g. the Academic Board of RCSLT or the Education and Research Board at COT.

Accreditation and validation

The Boards of the CPSM approve courses and examinations to ensure that graduates are fit to practise. Many professional organisations have a Joint Validation Committee, which oversees the joint work between the professional organisation and the CPSM's relevant Board to ensure that courses are validated.

In the past, many courses were delivered in NHS schools, attached to a hospital. Over the past few years, a steady wave of mergers and closures amongst these schools has taken place, together with a process of integration within higher education institutions. This occurred at a time when higher education institutions themselves were undergoing profound change, including a move from polytechnic to university status. Today, the vast majority of preregistration courses for care professionals takes place in the higher education setting.

Higher education institutions have to follow both internal and external quality processes before they can offer an education and training course. For example, the Higher Education Quality Council and the Higher Education Funding Council for England (and its counterparts in other areas of the UK) undertake audit and assessment activities.

Much of the work related to accreditation and validation of courses concerns quality assurance and monitoring, and changes to these are expected in the near future. There has been some criticism of the fairly onerous nature of quality-assurance processes for courses relating to care professionals delivered in the higher education sector. In the main, these have to satisfy the requirements of:

- the CPSM and the higher education funding councils (there is one such council for each of the four UK countries and also a similar structure for further education)
- the professional organisation
- very frequently, the higher education institution's own quality-control framework.

It can be argued that such complexity is, to a certain extent, unavoidable, given the vocational nature of education and training for a care profession. Nonetheless, some efforts are being made to streamline procedures.

The Higher Education Funding Council for England has co-ordinated a consultation project which has culminated in a report which proposes a single organisation at national level with responsibility for quality assurance in higher education institutions. This initiative would rely on an integration of quality-assurance processes to ensure that all requirements of the various parties are met, including those of what the report calls professional statutory organisations, and which include professional organisations. One chief aim would be to prevent duplication of effort or the placing of too onerous a demand on providers of education and training.

Wider role of professional organisations in education and training

The involvement of professional organisations in education and training matters does not limit itself to the accreditation and joint validation of preregistration courses. They accredit and jointly validate a whole range of courses at postgraduate/postregistration level for qualified professionals, such as postgraduate Diplomas or Master's degrees; they are also involved in education, training and development programmes for support workers, such as National Occupational Standards and National Vocational Qualifications.

In addition, professional organisations are often called upon in an advisory or consultation capacity when issues of relevance to therapists' and future therapists' education and training are raised nationally. For instance, many have provided input to the large-scale consultation exercise which led to the publication of the 'Dearing Review' (the report of the National Committee into Higher Education.) Many are also represented in the Health and Care Professions Education Forum, a organisation which was set up in 1989 to co-ordinate many education and training initiatives and whose scope extends beyond therapy professions, enjoying representation from midwives', health visitors' and Social Services organisations. Recently, a milestone in the Forum's activities has been the key contribution to the development and launch of National Occupational Standards for Health Promotion and Care.

Finally, much activity is taking place with many professional organisations around CPD and not just in therapy professional groups.

Definers of professional standards of practice and codes of conduct

How standards of practice and codes of conduct are developed

The definition of the professional standards of practice and the code of conduct, which set the framework for a professional group's behaviours at work and practices with patients and clients is, in many cases, the core function of a professional organisation. Often, the drawing up of these is the work of a specialist group within a professional organisation, e.g. the Professional Affairs Board. However, they are the object of much consultation, perhaps across an organisation's regional boards or committees, if these exist. In addition, special interest groups, which are groups of professionals set up under the aegis of a professional organisation to develop initiatives relevant to a particular client, care group or area of practice and management, may be involved in consultation.

Standards and codes of conduct are widely disseminated in publications, which are available for a fee (usually at a reduced rate for members of a professional organisation) or issued free. They evolve over time, as does therapeutic practice, and they aim to promote voluntary standards of behaviour and practice, acting as guidance rather than a definitive statement.

Professional standards of practice

There are many different professional standards of practice in place, as each professional organisation defines these for many different patients, clients or care groups. Standards are sometimes defined as models of care, or models of good or best practice. Some are the object of a manual or book. For example, the *Manual of Dietetic Practice* is published by the BDA and *Communicating Quality*, published by the RCSLT, is now in its second edition. Some are broad in scope (e.g. Professional Standards to be Achieved in Diagnostic Imaging, Radiotherapy and Oncology), whilst others are specific to the care provided in a particular situation (e.g. guidelines on acquired childhood aphasia published by the RCSLT).

Codes of conduct

The code of conduct drawn up by a professional organisation sets out guidelines, which provide a framework for the types of behaviour that therapists should adopt in their professional capacity. Examples of typical topics covered by a code of conduct include:

- codes of ethics in therapists' relations with patients and clients, e.g. the criteria in accepting referrals, or the rules governing advertising for professional services
- codes of professional and personal conduct, including the duty to maintain registration where applicable or the requirement to avoid behaviour which brings the profession into disrepute.

The future for therapists' professional organisations

Impact of the latest reforms

At the time of writing, the NHS and the care sector as a whole is experiencing another raft of profound changes. In December 1997, a government White Paper was published, setting out the broad framework for the *New NHS*, one which will continue its shift towards primary care provision, and where contracts and measures of performance against primarily financial targets are to be replaced by new models of care provision, commissioning and monitoring. These new models are still being developed, in the shape of pilots in the case of Health Action Zones and the emerging Primary Care Groups. Green Papers have been published on assessing the performance of NHS organisations and setting health promotion activities and strategies (*Our Healthier Nation*).

As well as impending legislative changes, other important developments are taking place. The review of the PSM Act is being mirrored in the nursing profession; a General Social Care Council is being set up to act as a professional organisation for social workers and others in Social

Services departments; and many changes are also afoot in the education sector with the recent government initiatives relating to lifelong learning, the response to the Dearing Review and the development of National Training Organisations. All of these developments are of relevance to therapists and their professional groups.

The intention of the government is to introduce change incrementally and the detailed shape of things to come is still unclear. However, the broad principles which emerge from the White Paper, the subsequent Green Papers and the other important developments which are taking place are clear. They can be summarised as follows:

- a reaffirmation of the centrality of primary care provision in the care sector as a whole
- a strong emphasis on partnerships and collaboration to improve health and offer care services involving the different partners in care at:
  - government department level; amongst the Department of Health (and equivalents in Wales, Scotland and Northern Ireland), Department of Social Security, and Department for Employment and Education
  - agency level; amongst NHS organisations, Social Services departments, general practitioners and voluntary sector organisations
  - organisational level, with collaboration rather than competition encouraged, and partnerships set to become stronger between professional organisations and higher education institutions
  - professional group level, with the promotion of interdisciplinary and multidisciplinary initiatives
- the notion of clinical governance: professional organisations, because of their roles as accrediting organisations and their involvement in the state registration of large numbers of professionals, will be playing a key part in this area.

Professional organisations and risk management

Another expression being used increasingly, and which is linked with the emerging notion of clinical governance, is that of risk management. Many Trusts have constituted risk-management groups that often encompass all aspects of the risk incurred by the Trust, including clinical risk. These groups can monitor and manage complaints and incidents; at a more strategic level, they might also examine the ways in which they can minimise risk for patients, clients and staff, perhaps by refocusing health and safety initiatives or seeking to remedy any deficiencies in staff training and development.

Professional organisations are potentially key players in risk management, for the same reasons as they might usefully be consulted on clinical governance issues: they have direct responsibilities in ensuring the fitness for practice of newly qualified staff through their accreditation and joint validation procedures with the higher education sector and the CPSM, where applicable. They can offer valuable advice to Trusts and other organisations employing therapists on subsequent training and development programmes. For example, many professional organisations recommend a period of one year for a newly qualified therapist to practise under supervision before they are deemed to be fully competent; many suggest frameworks for in-house training programmes for staff at different stages in their career, including return to practice after a career break. Finally, CPD is clearly a key element of risk management.

Summary

Professional organisations are an extremely diverse set of organisations, as evidenced by their different names, roles and functions, organisational structures and management arrangements. Nevertheless, they can be defined as offering the broad remit of representing their members (therapists) and contributing to the protection of the public, whilst also promoting practice development for the benefit of the care sector as a whole.

The services which professional organisations offer to their members include accreditation and validation of education and training courses, indemnity insurance, pay negotiations, other industrial relations services, professional standards of practice and codes of conduct, professional and career advice, and support and promotion of research and development

However, not all professional organisations undertake all of these activities. In addition, the CPSM confers the status of state registration for many (but not all) therapy professional groups. However, the Act which governs the CPSM is currently being reviewed and, as a result, the structure of the CPSM is expected to change. Amongst these changes are the protection of title for different therapy and other professional groups and the emergence of CPD, which may become a condition for the maintenance of registered status.

Trade union support, consisting largely of member support and representation in employment issues, is provided to therapists by their professional organisations in a variety of arrangements. Therapists can benefit from representation in disciplinary procedures, industrial tribunals and advice on a range of employment topics.

Specialist committees or boards within professional organisations have the remit to accredit and, jointly with the CPSM Boards, validate pre-registration courses which, upon satisfactory completion by students, will lead to their gaining state-registered status. The drawing up of codes of conduct and professional standards of practice is also a central function of professional organisations.

In the future, therapists and their professional organisations can expect to see many changes in the care sector with the introduction of new legislation and other important developments such as the review of the PSM Act and changes in the education sector. Specific areas of relevance to professional organisations will be the areas of CPD, and their links to corporate risk management and clinical governance. Therapists' professional organisations will be closely involved in the shaping of policies and practice in the UK care sector of the twenty-first century.

Chapter 10
Working Outside the National Health Service

Introduction

Most of this book has focused on the National Health Service (NHS) as the major working environment for young PAMs. Because of the good, all-round, basic experience that it provides in clinical practice, the NHS remains the recommended, initial, working environment for newly qualified therapists. However, more therapists now look to other employers or arrangements for opportunities to progress their career. The reasons for this vary. This chapter outlines the main ways in which therapists progress their clinical career, or widen their experience, outside the NHS.

The examples given in this chapter will be more or less relevant to different professions. For example, occupational therapists commonly work for Local Authorities but other professions rarely do so. Likewise, whilst private work for all professions is becoming more commonplace, Physiotherapists frequently work in private practice. All professions may have an interest in working abroad or in employment with a locum agency.

The chapter begins by outlining key aspects of working abroad. This is followed by information about working for private health-care providers and other employers, from both private and public sectors and locum or agency working. The chapter ends with a substantial section on private practice. The examples given in this chapter are not totally comprehensive and are not intended as such. In today's world, new and different opportunities for therapists continue to arise in many environments; this is likely to continue for some time.

Working abroad

As there is generally a global shortage of therapists, there are plenty of opportunities for PAMs wishing to work abroad. Many therapists who choose to work abroad do so in other English-speaking nations (mainly the USA, Canada, Australia, New Zealand and South Africa). For example, 50% of the members of the Chartered Society of Physiotherapy who currently work outside the UK are based in these countries. However, a variety of opportunities exists in a wide range of circumstances; from highly Westernised to developing countries, English-speaking to non-English-speaking countries, and fully paid employment to voluntary work.

Before work permits are granted to foreign therapists, each country's employment authority will wish to ensure that jobs offered to such therapists will not damage the employment prospects of its own nationals. Often, the types of position available in foreign countries are those less favoured by their own nationals, although the reasons for this may vary (e.g. geographic location, particular specialities or selected grades).

The admitting country will require documented evidence of therapists' qualifications and registration. Commonly, recruitment is organised through an agency familiar with the individual procedures of the recruiting country, but procedures may vary between different states of the same country, such as the USA. Obtaining authorisation or license to practise in foreign countries often requires entrees to sit examinations. The exact regulations vary for different professions and for each country or group of countries. Individual professional bodies should be consulted for information relevant to each profession and country or state.

The conduct of clinical practice in other countries is also likely to differ from that in the UK. Therapists working abroad must practise according to the rule of law and professional conduct of the country in which they are working. They must also be aware of the cultural differences that exist in other countries and respect them. Before accepting a job in another country, it is essential that therapists research and consider all major issues of clinical practice and daily life in their preferred country, to ensure that they can function in the environment they are likely to encounter. For example, there is a significant difference in the practice of respiratory care between the UK and USA: in the latter the majority of work is carried out by respiratory therapists, who form a separate professional group.

Working abroad brings a wealth of experience which adds not only to clinical skills, but also to personal growth and development. The extent to which this learning is recognised by prospective employers when therapists return to the UK is variable and can be reflected in the grade of post that returnees can expect to be offered. During periods of working abroad, therapists are advised to record in an appropriate format all learning as evidence of their continuing professional development (CPD).

Working for private health-care organisations

The most common private health-care organisation likely to employ PAMs is the private hospital. The number and range of PAMs staff employed by a private hospital are largely dependent on its size (which can vary from several to a few hundred beds) and the range of clinical specialities that it provides. Some private hospitals are restricted to surgical specialities (e.g. orthopaedics, gynaecology), whilst others provide a much wider range of medical and surgical services. Radiographers and physiotherapists have been employed in private hospitals for many years. More recently, with increasing emphasis on multidisciplinary working, occupational therapists and speech and language therapists have also been employed. Other professional groups such as dietitians and clinical psychologists may also be employed on an ad hoc, sessional or reduced time basis.

The terms and conditions of employment of private health-care providers may vary considerably from those considered as standard within the NHS. These include such issues as salary, entitlement to holiday, sickness and maternity leave, and pension schemes. There may be scope for negotiation within and between certain parameters. Positions with private organisations may also offer benefits which are not available within the NHS (e.g. bonus schemes, private health cover and health screening).

There are also some different expectations of therapists working in private hospitals. Firstly, patients' expectations of the care they receive are high; thus, private organisations pay significant attention to ensuring that high standards are consistently achieved in all aspects of care. Quality-control initiatives, including those which bring external accreditation (e.g. Kings Fund, Investors in People, Charter Mark), are an important part of the organisation. Therapists working in private hospitals may also have responsibilities associated with the financial aspects of their service. Private patients must pay for their treatments, often via insurance schemes, and there will be defined procedures for charging and billing. In some cases these procedures may affect the clinical situation and the treatment plan drawn up between the therapist and patient. For example, a patient may only be able to afford to pay for a fixed or small number of treatment sessions. Many insurance companies also restrict the number of treatment sessions allowed, although therapists can sometimes negotiate an extension to standard arrangements.

PAMs may also find work opportunities in a range of other private health-care organisations. These include private rehabilitation centres (e.g. specialist units such as those for head injury or children), nursing, residential or care homes and hospices. The principles given above for private hospitals also apply in these environments.

Working for locum agencies

Many therapists work for a locum agency at some stage in their career and for a range of reasons; however, such an arrangement is usually short term or temporary. Today, there is a wide range of locum agencies. Many deal with a number of PAMs, whilst some specialise in a particular profession; others may focus on a particular geographical area.

Most locum positions are required for and thus offered as a fixed-term arrangement, from a few days to a number of weeks or even months. Organisations requiring locum staff subcontract the therapist from the agency, and the agency employs the therapist. Traditionally, therapists employed as locums received a higher rate of pay but little else from the employing agency: employees received no pay for sickness absence, study leave, etc. This is gradually changing, with some agencies offering additional perks such as low-cost car lease and loyalty bonus schemes. Many are now keen to assist locum therapists in CPD.

It is worth understanding the requirements of services for locum staff. Locum therapists are often required to meet service pressures where there is an unfilled vacancy or short-term funding has been made available to deal with particular issues (e.g. winter pressures). The costs of locum staff are high (about twice the cost of regular employees) and managers expect locum therapists to undertake clinical work; they may not allocate time for in-service training or similar activities. Thus, therapists undertaking locum work should not expect the entitlements of an organisation's own employees.

Whilst locum work provides a higher level of pay, this may come at a cost. Continual locum work may not provide, and does not guarantee, a level of experience and training which prepares new graduate therapists for their future career.

Working for other employers

In addition to those described previously, there is a number of organisations that commonly employ therapists and offer a variety of career options.

Other public sector

Local Authorities and Social Services departments

Local authorities frequently employ occupational therapists to provide therapy or to work with Housing Departments in the provision of specialist equipment or housing adaptations. Local Authorities have their own terms and conditions of employment.

Armed forces

The UK's armed forces have their own health service, including their own hospitals, and opportunities exist for all PAMs to work in this environment.

Charitable organisations

Registered charities also employ therapists in a number of ways: as advisors, to provide education and training for their members or to provide therapy for their patient group. Many of these positions are offered on a part-time or sessional basis.

Commercial companies

Some large commercial companies employ therapists in an advisory role or to provide a treatment service for their employees. Examples include undertaking risk or ergonomic assessments in the workplace or physiotherapy treatment to facilitate return to work. Some public-sector services, such as the police, also offer such opportunities. PAMs may find that their qualifications, training and experience lend themselves to other related fields, such as sports medicine for physiotherapists or food technology for dietitians.

Private practice

Many PAMs, as a result of the type of service and treatment that they provide, are able to undertake private practice. Many do so on an ad hoc, informal or part-time basis. However, increasing numbers of PAMs now seek full-time independent practice as their chosen work environment. This usually involves being self-employed and responsible for all aspects of the therapy service, usually in an out-patient setting.

Full-time private practice involves a range of activities including establishing the practice, delivering the clinical service, management of the practice and generation of sufficient work to secure an adequate income. Success in these activities generally requires some previous managerial experience.

The following paragraphs provide information on the basic requirements for full-time private practice. Whilst there are many ways in which to enter private practice, the text illustrates the scenario of the self-employed practitioner in sole practice.

Considering private practice

There are several important differences between private practice and working for an employer (Table 10.1). It is generally inadvisable for those in poor health to enter self-employed practice.

Table 10.1 Key differences between private practice and working for an employer

	NHS (as example of employer)	Private practice
National Insurance	NI contributions and income tax (PAYE) deducted at source	Must organise own payment of NI contributions. Different benefits. Tax on profits (Schedule D)
Pension	Optional if working 18–36 h per week; compulsory if > 36 h	Must set up own self-employment pension scheme
Holiday pay	Automatic	Must fund own holiday absence or pay locums
Sickness	Paid sick leave (depending on length of service)	Must arrange insurance cover for loss of earnings
Income	Known	Variable
Uniform	Provided or an allowance paid	Own choice and expense
Contact with colleagues	Constant	Potentially isolated; contact is dependent on own effort
Hours of work	Set plus emergency duty	According to workload
Equipment	Purchased and serviced by employer	Must arrange and take responsibility for own purchase and maintenance
Liability insurance	NHS has vicarious liability as employer	Own responsibility
Administration	Partial responsibility	Total responsibility
Further training	May be provided and paid for	At own responsibility and expense

Private practice is not for the newly qualified. Although a minimum of 2 years' postqualification experience is essential, it is advisable to have 5 years of general experience covering the broad scope of practice before setting up in full-time practice.

Starting a private practice

Location

Starting a private practice may mean buying or leasing business premises, establishing a practice as part of a home, working with other established practitioners in existing premises or undertaking domiciliary practice where no premises are required. The location of the practice is crucial: the best location is where the greatest number of patient opportunities exists. Market research should be undertaken, encompassing the size and economy of the local community, adequacy of existing therapy services (NHS and private), alternative therapies, adequate referral sources and possible demand for the specific skills of the therapist.

If choosing to move to an area to establish a practice, then the chosen community must also be evaluated from a personal and family perspective. Establishing a private practice usually requires long and unsociable hours of work, which can create family pressures and reduce personal leisure time.

Obtaining a practice

The following types of business relationship or set-up are open to the private practitioner.

- *A sole practitioner* is responsible for all aspects of the service and is always self-employed.
- *Assistant or locum*: one of the least expensive ways of entering private practice is to work within an established practice. This can be achieved either as a self-employed practitioner who contracts their services to an existing practice or as an employee of the practice. Therapists considering such a position should ensure that they receive a proper employment agreement with the practice owner which sets out employment terms and conditions.
- *Associate, partner or director in an existing practice*: a proper agreement is essential, and legal and financial advice should always be sought from a solicitor or an accountant before a formal agreement is signed.

A number of issues associated with establishing a new practice can be overcome by purchasing an existing practice. These include:

- establishing a patient caseload
- employing staff
- building relationships with referral sources
- establishing an income.

The purchase itself is often a complex process and appropriate legal and financial advice should always be sought. It may be useful to consider the following questions.

- Why is the practice for sale?
- What are the assets of the practice?
- What is the condition of the equipment?
- What sort of contacts are in place with existing staff?
- Will the staff remain?
- Will the practice principal work with you to introduce you to the practice?
- What sort of competition is there?
- What is the financial outlook for the practice?
- How much should you pay?
- Is there a value for 'good will'?

Equipping and staffing the practice

Once the research and analysis outlined above have been undertaken it should be possible to list the equipment necessary to deliver the desired service. This should include not only clinical equipment, but furniture for waiting and office areas, computers and transport, if a domiciliary service is to be provided. As a rough guide, a new practice could cost in the region of £10,000 (excluding premises and building alternations) to equip fully. Equipment can be bought second-hand, but electrical equipment should have a maintenance certificate and be checked by a suitably qualified electrical engineer. Equipment can also be leased.

Additional therapists or administrative staff may be needed. The success of the practice will largely be determined by the calibre and capabilities of its staff. It is vital to recruit suitable personnel, establish appropriate employment contracts and understand staff management issues.

Financial aspects of practice

Even when detailed planning has been undertaken, there will always be an element of financial risk when establishing a private practice. This risk can be lessened and the probability of success increased if the professional goals and financial position of the business are properly understood.

Perhaps the most important issue to understand is the break-even point of the practice. This activity involves an analysis of fixed and variable costs together with expected income. From this, a clear picture is developed of how many hours (and therefore how many patients) the practice must generate to produce the income required to cover its costs. Advice should be taken from an accountant to ensure a thorough understanding of the financial situation.

Income generation is perhaps best understood by recognising that treatment is 'free' until it is paid for, and that the contract within a private practice is always between a patient who is responsible for payment and the therapist who is responsible for delivering appropriate treatment. Income is often delayed when medical insurance companies reimburse the patient or the practice and this must be taken into account when anticipating income. Accurate and thorough records of the practice's financial position must be kept to evaluate the performance of the practice and for audit purposes.

Insurance

The insurance needs of the practice should be determined by comprehensive risk assessment. Depending on the nature of the practice and the personal needs of the practice owner, adequate levels of insurance for all or some of the following may be necessary:

- professional liability insurance
- public liability insurance
- all-risks practice insurance
- employer's insurance
- permanent heath insurance
- life insurance
- mortgage insurance
- additional car insurance where patients or equipment are transported.

The list is not exhaustive but must be tailored to suit practice needs.

Legal aspects of practice

Key legal aspects of practice encompass both clinical and business activities.

- *Clinical*: adequate patient records must be kept. When medical malpractice cases occur, they are most effectively defended when medical records support the therapist's position that safe, effective, professional treatment was administered. Clinical records must be stored in accordance with good practice and legal requirements. Access to clinical records must be available in accordance with the law (see Chapter 6). Licensing by Local Authorities and meeting specific health and safety regulations may be required for specific clinical modalities such as acupuncture or the use of lasers.
- *Business*: health and safety law applies to clinic facilities even when they are part of a home. Financial records are necessary to provide an analysis for the purposes of taxation. It is also essential to find out whether the local authority requires the premises to be licensed (this is variable) or planning permission for change of use; general advice on local rules and by-laws is also helpful.

Managerial functions in private practice

In single-handed practice, management is the responsibility of the practice principal. In partnerships and other working relationships, managerial responsibilities are often shared. Key function at the start-up phase include:

- objective setting
- planning
- establishment of practice policies and procedures
- organisation
- communication
- budget setting
- practice review.

Marketing

Marketing is essential in the initial and ongoing development of a private practice. Marketing aims to position the practice and its services within the community in a manner that identifies and fulfils an unsatisfied patient need. A practice will thus aim to offer therapy services that are either unavailable or available to an unsatisfactory level in a community.

The health-care marketplace is constantly evolving in response to economic pressures and the strategies of successive governments. Successful private practitioners must understand this evolution as it occurs and ensure that their practices adapt as necessary.

Quality and price

Despite tight controls over the costs of health care in the NHS and private sector, there remains a chronic shortage of funds in both. Neither public taxation nor increases in subscription levels by medical insurance companies provide sufficient resources for the demand for health care today. This situation is certain to continue. Thus, the focus of both the private sector and the Government is on maximising the use of available funds by:

- increasing operational efficiency
- improving (and measuring) outcome via clinical and cost-effective practice
- raising quality standards.

Both private- and public-sector purchasers demand a quality service at a competitive price. Private practices must consider this when setting prices for their services, along with the prices and quality of services provided by their competitors.

Accreditation will become increasingly important for quality assurance within private practices over the coming years.

Private practice customers

There are three principal sources of patients for a private practice.

- *Patients with private health insurance cover*: these can represent an important proportion of workload for private practices. Any changes to procedures or approach by the large insurers can thus have a serious impact on the practice.
- *Patients referred by general practitioners (GPs)*: a small percentage of patients in the average practice are individuals who have been referred directly by their GP. Thus, it can be beneficial knowing, and being known to, local GP practices. A number of trends and factors may impact on GP referrals:
  - GPs may already have contracts with other therapists
  - GPs are increasingly employing their own therapist
  - GPs are becoming more open to alternative and complementary therapies
  - the latest NHS reforms will remove GP fundholding and change contracting arrangements which may tend to route contracts back into the NHS.
- *Self-referral*: The public are becoming increasingly well informed about the treatments available to help them and frequently self-refer for private therapy. All referrers and patients look for a service which offers:
  - quick appointments at convenient times
  - a holistic approach to the problem, including education and preventive advice
  - specialist expertise
  - individual attention and treatment.

There are many opportunities for therapists to move into private or independent practice, whether treating an occasional patient or setting up in full-time practice.

Consultation with appropriate professionals, such as accountants, bank managers, solicitors, surveyors and professional bodies, will provide valuable advice to the prospective private practitioner. The issues highlighted above will require careful consideration before therapists embark on a significant private practice career.

Summary

This chapter has described a number of alternative employment or career opportunities available to therapists. It should be remembered that the examples given are more or less relevant to different professions. The chapter has outlined key aspects of working abroad, working for private health-care providers, other private- or public-sector organisations, and locum or agency working; there is a substantial section on private practice.

Owing to its size as an employer, the working arrangements within the NHS tend to be a benchmark against which PAMs' employment terms and conditions in other environments are compared. Therapists considering working outside the NHS should investigate differences in their proposed new employment and consider implications for short- and long-term career prospects before accepting a position.

The examples given in the chapter are not totally comprehensive and are not intended as such. In today's world, new and different opportunities for therapists continue to arise in many environments and this is likely to continue for some time.

Index